Llyfrgell Sir POWYS County Library
Llandrindod Wells LD1 5LD
www.powys.gov.uk/libraries

Barcode No. ..00425182.............   Class No. ....613.265....

BAILEY, Christine
The raw food diet

This book must be returned by the last date stamped above.
Rhaid dychwelyd y llyfr hwn erbyn y dyddiad diwethaf a stampiwyd uchod.

A charge will be made for any lost, damaged or overdue books.
Codir tâl os bydd llyfr wedi ei golli neu ei ni weidio neu heb ei ddychwelyd
mewn pryd.

D0177354

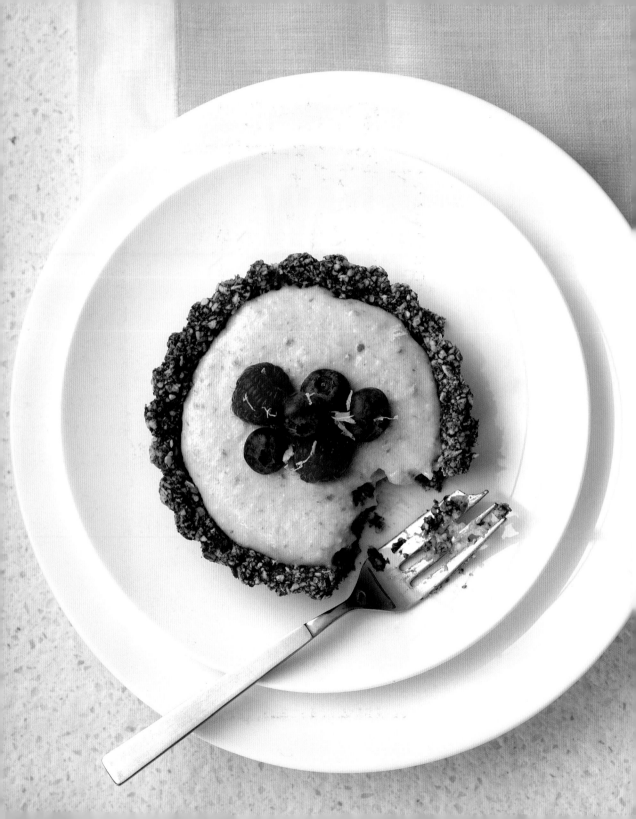

THE RAW FOOD DIET

THE HEALTHY WAY TO GET THE SHAPE YOU WANT

CHRISTINE BAILEY

DUNCAN BAIRD PUBLISHERS

LONDON

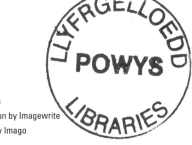

The Raw Food Diet
Christine Bailey

First published in the United Kingdom and Ireland
in 2012 by
Duncan Baird Publishers Ltd
Sixth Floor, Castle House
75–76 Wells Street
London W1T 3QH

Conceived, created and designed by
Duncan Baird Publishers

Managing Editor: Grace Cheetham
Editors: Helen Brocklehurst, Alison Bolus
Managing Designer: Manisha Patel
Designer: Gail Jones
Production: Uzma Taj
Commissioned Photography: Toby Scott
Food Stylists: Jayne Cross, Denise Smart
Prop Stylist: Tamsin Weston

British Library Cataloguing-in-Publication Data:
A CIP record for this book is available from the
British Library

ISBN: 978-1-84483-994-0
1 3 5 7 9 10 8 6 4 2

Typeset in Univers
Colour reproduction by Imagewrite
Printed in China by Imago

Publisher's note
The information in this book is not intended as a
substitute for professional medical advice and treatment.
The information and recipes are unsuitable if you are
pregnant or lactating; are under the age of 18; are
scheduled for or have just had surgery; are diabetic or
have metabolic syndrome, Wilson's disease or AIDS; or
suffer from any eating disorder. If you have any special
dietary requirements or other medical conditions, it is
recommended that you consult a medical professional
before following any of the information or recipes
contained in this book. Duncan Baird Publishers, or any
other persons who have been involved in working on this
publication, cannot accept responsibility for any errors
or omissions, inadvertent or not, that may be found in the
recipes or text, nor for any problems that may arise as a
result of preparing one of these recipes or following the
advice contained in this work.

Notes on the recipes
Unless otherwise stated:
Use medium fruit and vegetables
Use fresh ingredients, including herbs and chillies
Do not mix metric and imperial measurements
1 tsp = 5ml 1 tbsp = 15ml 1 cup = 250ml

Author's acknowledgments
My thanks to Grace and Alison at DBP for their ongoing
support and guidance in writing this book. A special
thanks to my patient, supportive husband and my three
fantastic children, Nathan, Isaac and Simeon, for trying
out every recipe and giving such wonderful feedback
and encouragement.

I have used an Excaliber dehydrator for all the recipes in
this book and have used Teflex non-stick sheets.

contents

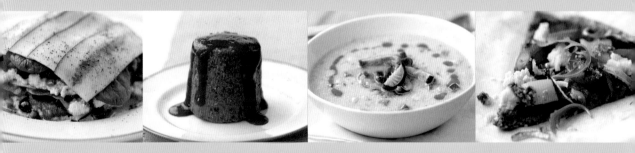

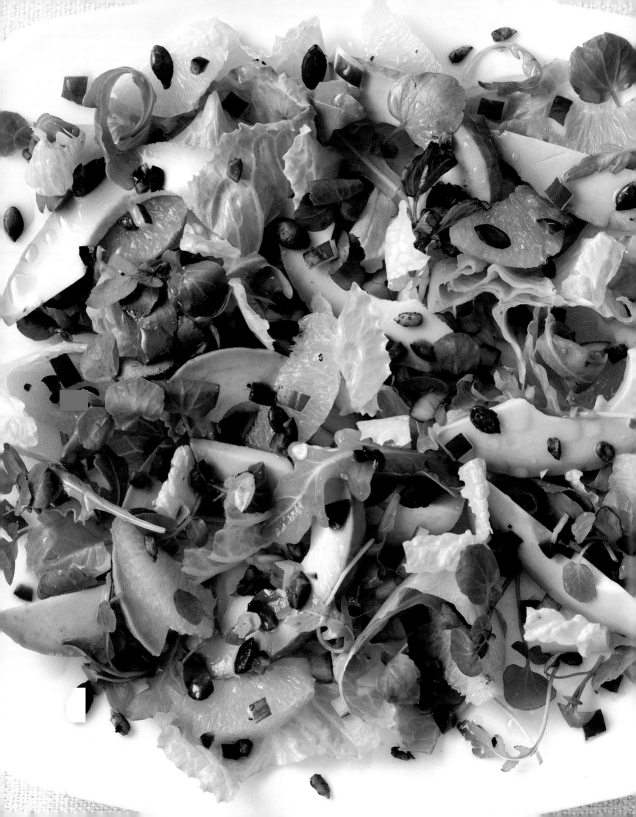

introduction

If you want to lose weight and enjoy a healthier, more vibrant life, then *The Raw Food Diet* is for you. Packed with an amazing array of delicious recipes, this book will show you how easy it is to include more raw foods in your diet, and, by doing so, help you achieve a slimmer, younger-looking body with renewed energy and vitality.

Whether you just want to lose a bit of weight or are struggling with long-term weight and health issues, this raw food diet will enable you to achieve your maximum weight loss with minimum effort, and transform your health for good. You can choose the Raw Food Weekend Blitz Diet, the Raw Food Week Diet or the Raw for Life Diet, and there is no need to count calories or carbs. Instead, this programme is all about high-quality, nutrient-dense foods to nourish your body and enable it to function optimally. Raw foods will not only satisfy your appetite and stabilize blood sugar levels, but also energize you and cleanse your body to leave you feeling amazing.

< Avocado, Citrus and Spiced Seed Salad with Olive Vinaigrette (page 46)

why raw food?

So what is raw food? Simply put, it is food that has not been heated to above 47.7°C/118°F. Typically, it is pure, unadulterated, whole food that is rich in vitamins, minerals, enzymes and phytonutrients (specific nutrients found in plants).

The term "living foods" generally refers to foods that are still alive and growing, in addition to living greens such as wheatgrass and sunflower greens. A raw food diet is therefore one that is based around plenty of vegetables (especially green leafy vegetables), fruit and nuts. It does not include any processed or refined foods. Liquids are also an essential component of the diet in the form of water, fresh juices, herbal infusions, nut milks and smoothies.

losing weight the raw food way

So how does eating more raw food encourage weight loss and renew energy? Firstly, raw foods such as vegetables, herbs and fruits are incredibly nutrient dense and energizing, possessing many healing and health-promoting properties. Partly, this is due to their phytochemical content. Phytochemicals are natural bioactive substances present in plant foods and they are found in their highest quantities in raw, freshly harvested plants. When food is processed and/or heated to temperatures of 47.7°C/118°F and above, many of the natural enzymes, phytonutrients and essential nutrients are destroyed or are made less bio-available. Cooking can also produce unnatural chemical substances, the processing of which places additional strain on the body's detoxification organs, such as the liver, gut and kidneys.

Secondly, enzymes are required for numerous chemical and metabolic processes in our bodies, including energy production and detoxification. By simply incorporating more raw food in your diet you are providing your body with an abundance of essential enzymes, nutrients and fibre, all of which are needed for the body to process food,

the benefits of the raw food diet

Supercharge your diet with amazing cleansing and rejuvenating raw food. Include more raw food in your diet and experience a range of benefits:

- Lose weight
- Improve digestion
- Improve immune function – fewer colds and infections
- Have a clearer, more radiant complexion and healthier hair
- Increase energy and vitality
- Reduce fluid retention and bloating
- Improve mental clarity
- Get relief from allergies
- Improve quality of sleep
- Reduce the risk of heart disease, diabetes and other chronic conditions

detoxify, create energy and perform at its optimum. They enable your body to break down foods more effectively and absorb optimum nutrients for every cell in your body, and they aid the elimination of waste and toxins. Helping the body detoxify is essential for weight loss. When our liver is overworked and we can't detoxify effectively, waste products and toxins will be stored in our fat cells – so the more toxins that are in our bodies, the more fat cells that are needed, and the harder it is to lose weight. It can also lead to inflammation, which can damage tissues and accelerate the signs of ageing. And if the body is not digesting and absorbing foods properly, you can end up starved of essential nutrients and feeling tired and fatigued. A raw food diet, therefore, works in many ways to improve your health: on the one hand, you are providing your body with nutrients to help it function more effectively and clean itself, while on the other hand you are avoiding foods that diminish the efficiency of both nutrient absorption and detoxification.

By nourishing the liver with raw foods, you also enable it to carry out other important tasks more effectively, such as balancing blood sugar, reducing cravings, eliminating excess hormones and producing bile to break down fats and keep cholesterol levels healthy. As a bonus, raw foods are also hydrating and satiating, which means they enable you to feel fuller for longer while keeping energy levels high.

Fruit and vegetables, especially raw leafy greens, which are full of chlorophyll, have the added benefit of being incredibly alkalizing. If you eat cooked, processed foods and animal products, this increases the body's acidity. Too many acid-forming foods can promote inflammation, lower immune function and reduce levels of alkaline minerals, such as calcium and magnesium. By nourishing the body with alkalizing foods each day, you help to restore your body's pH balance, enabling it to heal and regenerate itself. In fact, just by eating raw foods you are literally supercharging your body with optimum nutrition to help rejuvenate it and promote vibrant health. As it rejuvenates you, you will find yourself losing excess weight more easily and so feeling lighter, leaner and energized.

A raw food diet does not necessarily mean exclusively 100% raw. For some people a raw food diet means eating raw food during the day and then having a cooked meal in the evening, so around 50% raw. For others it may mean 80% raw and 20% cooked in a day. The key is to find what works for you. Even if you think you have a healthy diet, you are probably eating only about 20–25% raw food. By including more raw food into your diet, you are likely to experience a significant difference to your health and achieve your weight loss.

An easy way to start increasing your intake of raw, nutritious foods is to begin the day with a green smoothie or raw juice (see page 22) These are hydrating and energizing as well as being gentle on the digestive system. Once you have tried that, you could then start experimenting with some of the delicious raw salads and soups provided in this book.

about the raw food diet programme

The book is separated into three chapters: the Raw Food Weekend Blitz Diet; the Raw Food Week Diet; and the Raw For Life Diet. Each of these chapters contains a programme that includes helpful information and example diet plans, plus raw food recipes specially designed to help you lose weight, support digestive and liver health, and also supercharge your energy levels.

The Raw Food Weekend Blitz Diet chapter includes an intensive two-and-a-half-day programme incorporating three raw food meals and snacks to keep your metabolism high, enabling you to lose weight fast. The focus is on simple, light recipes to support cleansing and rejuvenation. This is a great plan to start with if you are new to eating raw food, looking for a short-term cleanse, or just want to lighten up and lose a little weight.

The Raw Food Week Diet chapter contains a seven-day programme comprising raw meals and snacks to help stabilize blood sugar levels and curb cravings, while encouraging detoxification to assist longer-term weight loss. Some of the recipes require a little more preparation than the Weekend Blitz, enabling you to experience a greater variety of raw foods and dishes. The emphasis is on recipes that include easy-to-find ingredients and nutrient-dense foods that satisfy and provide the body with essential nutrients to supercharge energy levels and assist with weight loss.

The Raw for Life Diet chapter focuses on incorporating a greater range of fresh, nutritious dishes into your everyday life, whether you are looking to move to a largely raw diet or just wishing to adopt healthier recipes to eat alongside your cooked dishes. By gradually increasing the amount of raw food you include in your diet, you will flood your body with the vitamins, minerals and enzymes your body needs to function more optimally. This can bring greater vitality to your life and help you to maintain a lean, healthy body. Even if you have been eating raw food for a while, you will find many new recipes to try in this chapter. There are also recipes that are ideal for entertaining or as an occasional treat.

starting in the raw

If you are new to eating raw food, then it is recommended that you gradually increase the amount of raw food in your diet before starting one of the programmes in this book. Begin the day with one of the freshly pressed juices or smoothies, followed by a raw breakfast option. Look through the recipes in this book and select a couple that appeal to you. Then look to include a large raw salad during the day using one of the recipes in this book. Make sure you have a variety of ingredients, including green leafy vegetables, herbs, seeds, nuts, sea vegetables and a nutrient-rich dressing. Do this for at least a week before starting the Raw Food Weekend plan. By gradually making changes to your diet, you are more likely to experience longer-lasting weight loss and improved health. For this reason, it is also important that you start to cut out certain foods and drinks from your diet, including gluten grains, dairy, refined carbohydrates (sugary foods, drinks and processed foods), caffeine, fizzy drinks, trans and hydrogenated fats, meat and processed meat products.

Once you have completed the Raw Food Weekend, you can progress to the Raw Food Week programme. This is designed to help the body cleanse itself of waste and toxins and for you to experience not only noticeable weight loss but also renewed energy and vitality. After the Raw Food Week programme, you can either continue with this eating plan or focus on increasing your consumption of raw foods using the additional recipes in the Raw for Life Diet section. Whether you plan to follow one of the programmes or devise your own using the recipes in the book, the more you incorporate raw, fresh food in your diet, the better you will look and feel, and the easier you will find it to achieve a healthy weight. Please note that if you have any long-term health problems or medical conditions, it is always advised that you consult with a suitably qualified medical practitioner before embarking on any new diet plan.

Remember, you don't have to eat solely raw food to enjoy the recipes in this book — they are suitable for everyone and are incredibly nutritious. They are also beneficial for those on special diets needing to avoid gluten, eggs, dairy or processed foods and additives. The recipes are simple and nourishing; many can also be prepared in advance.

For optimal health and weight loss, the recipes in this book focus on low glycemic index foods, keeping sweeteners to a minimum. Sugar in all its forms is broken down by the body into glucose. Sudden rises in glucose trigger the production of insulin, which in turn converts glucose into fat and ultimately weight gain. Therefore, if you want to lose weight it is important to minimize these insulin spikes by basing your diet around foods that are broken down slowly by the body (low glycemic index foods). Low glycemic sweeteners that are recommended in the recipes include stevia, yacon syrup, coconut nectar and xylitol (see page 17). While xylitol is not a raw ingredient, it is a natural, low glycemic sweetener, readily available, which does not impact on blood sugar levels. Agave nectar is not recommended due to its high fructose content. Flower pollen has been used in

a couple of the recipes for its protein, energy and immune-enhancing properties. In other recipes, fresh fruit or dried fruit is used to provide sweetness, while also adding fibre and additional nutrients.

If you suffer with digestive difficulties it is suggested that you eat fruit separately from other foods – at least half an hour before consuming your next meal. This is because fruit digests much more quickly than fats, proteins and starches. Fruit can, however, mix well with greens, so these can be incorporated together in drinks and salads. Avoid drinking at mealtimes, as this dilutes digestive juices. It is also helpful to eat your evening meal early to give your digestive system time to process food before bedtime. Eating too late can lead to gas, bloating and a heavy feeling all night. Eating less in the evening will also help you wake up feeling lighter and more vibrant too. To keep your blood sugar levels balanced through the day, include a few protein-rich snacks, such as sprouted seeds, pâtés and dips, nuts and seeds, using the recipes in this book, or drink a smoothie or some nut milk.

nutritional considerations

Whichever programme you follow, optimize your health by eating some superfoods and taking supplements. Many of the superfoods are included in the recipes, but it is suggested that you supplement daily with a high-quality multivitamin and mineral formula, and a vitamin B complex formula that includes B12. To optimize essential fats in the body, include omega-3-rich foods daily, such as chia seeds, flaxseeds, walnuts, hemp seeds and leafy greens, and supplement with an omega-3 formula supplying EPA and DHA. Modern lifestyles make it difficult to get adequate vitamin D from sunshine-based synthesis, especially in cold climates, and a vegan-based diet is more likely to be deficient. Daily vegan vitamin D supplements are recommended. Choline is important for certain brain functions and lipid metabolism, and can be low in vegan diets. Lecithin powders are a useful source of choline. You should also take a digestive enzyme formula with each meal to assist in digestion. Here are some useful raw superfoods that you should stock up on:

Acai and other berry powders
Nutritionally, acai is considered a true antioxidant powerhouse, containing a range of phytonutrients such as polyphenols and flavonoids. It is also rich in healthy monounsaturated and polyunsaturated fatty acids. Processed into powders, these are an easy way to boost the nutrition of recipes and drinks.

Raw cacao powder Derived from cold-pressed cacao beans, it is packed with antioxidants (flavanols and polyphenols) and a concentrated source of nutrients, especially magnesium, and mood-boosting tryptophan and phenylethylamine. The powder and nibs also provide a useful source of dietary fibre and iron.

Flower pollen This is a complete superfood containing an incredible array of vitamins, minerals, amino acids and enzymes. It is thought to promote the growth of friendly bacteria in the intestine and thereby support the immune system. Being particularly rich in folic acid and the other B group vitamins, it is important for energy production. It is also a useful source of the antioxidant rutin – known to help strengthen capillaries, support blood vessels and enhance circulation.

Lucuma powder A nutrient-dense fruit from Peru, lucuma is traditionally used in ice creams and desserts. With a maple syrup flavour, it is a useful natural sweetener. It also provides plenty of fibre, vitamins and minerals, including beta-carotene, niacin (vitamin B3) and iron.

Maca powder A Peruvian root vegetable commonly found in a powdered form and rich in protein, iron and calcium. It is naturally sweet and delicious added to drinks, cakes and desserts. It is renowned as a hormone balancer, an aphrodisiac and an adaptogen, supporting the adrenal glands and increasing energy levels.

Mesquite powder This is produced from the seed-pods of the mesquite tree. It is high in protein and minerals, such as calcium, magnesium, potassium, iron and zinc. You can also use it to replace the flour in cakes, cookies and pastry. Lower on the glycemic index than most other sweeteners, it can help to regulate blood sugar and curb appetite. With a toffee-like flavour, it is a useful sweetener in smoothies and desserts.

Green superfood powders such as chlorella, Klamath lake blue green algae, spirulina, barley grass and wheatgrass cleanse and alkalize, and are packed with protein, vitamins and minerals. Take 1 tsp daily or add to drinks or food.

Stevia This is a natural low glycemic, zero-calorie sweetener that does not affect blood sugar levels. At 300 times sweeter than sugar, a little goes a long way.

Yacon syrup Extracted from an Andean plant, yacon is a popular low-calorie low glycemic index sweetener. Rich in prebiotic inulin, it is a complex sugar that can help digestive health and promote the growth of healthy bacteria in the gut. It tastes a little like caramel and molasses. Use it in recipes as you would honey.

the raw food larder

The recipes in this book focus on using nutritient-dense raw foods. I recommend choosing as much organic produce as you can afford and ensuring it is as fresh as possible for maximum benefits. The majority of the ingredients used in this book can be bought from supermarkets, farmers markets and good independent health shops. They are also available from online suppliers. Not all of the ingredients used in the recipes are 100% raw, such as xylitol or tamari soy sauce, but these are healthy, nutritious additions to recipes for enhanced flavour and texture. Here's what you will need:

Fresh fruits and vegetables, frozen fruit

Ready-sprouted seeds and beans or beans/seeds to sprout yourself.

Frozen wheatgrass juice This can be purchased in ice cube trays ready for using in juice and smoothie recipes and for drinking as a "shot". This is particularly useful if you do not have a juicer or do not have the time to juice and grow your own wheatgrass. Trays of fresh wheatgrass and other "living grasses", such as barley grass, can also be bought if you do not wish to grow them yourself but want a ready supply to juice. You will, however, need to check that your juicer is robust enough to juice wheatgrass.

Nuts Pine nuts, cashews, walnuts, pecans, almonds, hazelnuts, macadamia nuts. Also worth trying are nut butters, coconut flakes, desiccated coconut and coconut water.

Seeds Pumpkin, sunflower and sesame seeds, shelled hemp seeds, tahini, ground and whole flaxseeds, buckwheat groats, chia and quinoa. Packed with essential fats, protein, vitamins and minerals, these are nourishing and energizing. Try including at least 1 tbsp daily in dishes, drinks or as a part of breakfast, with a glass of water. Chia seeds are often made into a gel to add to smoothies, soups, jellies and sauces. Put 2 tbsp into 250ml/9fl oz/ 1 cup liquid and stir occasionally for 15–20 minutes. Refrigerate for up to a week.

Oils Coconut butter (also called coconut oil), flaxseed and hemp oils, and extra virgin olive oil. For the best quality, choose cold-pressed oils, preferably organic. To melt coconut butter, place in a bowl over hot water for 5 minutes or in a dehydrator for 5–10 minutes.

Sea vegetables, including kelp noodles, nori sheets and sea vegetable salad mix. Sea vegetables are bought dried and are used to enhance dishes, such as salads, wraps and raw soups and sauces. They are often soaked before using.

Flavourings Himalayan sea salt, or Celtic salt, garlic salt, freshly ground black pepper, nutritional yeast flakes (dried, not raw), onion powder, vanilla extract, spices and dried herbs, fresh herbs, garlic and chillies add flavour to dishes. Although sea salts can contain traces of minerals, they are essentially still sodium chloride (salt), so add as minimally as possible. Other flavourings and condiments that you want to add should always be used in moderation.

Condiments Cider vinegar, rice, balsamic and red wine vinegars, tamari soy sauce, white miso paste, marinated sun-dried tomatoes, mustard and olives.

Sweeteners Xylitol (not raw), flower pollen, coconut nectar, yacon syrup, stevia, lucuma, mesquite, maca powder and any dried fruit. Dates are commonly used as a sweetener in recipes – often mixed into a paste with a little water. They also make a useful binder in pastry, cakes and cookies. Dates and other dried fruit, however, are high on the glycaemic index and contain varying amounts of glucose, fructose and sucrose. They should, therefore, be used sparingly in your raw food diet.

Xylitol Although it is not raw, xylitol is an ideal healthy sweetener to use in recipes. With 40% fewer calories than sugar and a low glycaemic index, it has minimal impact on blood sugar levels, which makes it ideal as part of a weight-loss programme. It also helps to maintain healthy teeth.

the raw food kitchen

A raw food diet does not have to mean expensive equipment and gadgets. You can start with just a few basic items and gradually build up according to the type of recipes you like to eat. Here are a few key items that will make your life easier and simpler, saving you time in the kitchen:

Food processor Perfect for blending ingredients, as well as chopping, slicing and grating with ease. If you can afford it, choose a robust, durable model with a range of grating and slicing options.

Blender A blender is perfect for making raw food: pulverizing nuts and seeds and making nut milks, raw cheese, smoothies, soups, dips and sauces with ease. It is also particularly useful for making nut flours, which are often used as the basis of raw crackers, bars and desserts. It is also useful for making instant ice creams and sorbets. If you want to crush ice, too, get a heavy-duty model.

Juicer A couple of recipes call for juicing fruit and vegetables. Choose a model that is robust enough to juice a range of vegetables, including leafy greens. A masticating juicer is ideal as it can handle a greater range of fruits and vegetables and is efficient at extracting the nutrients.

Nut milk bag A sturdy, lightweight nylon mesh bag that can be used repeatedly to make nut milk. They often have a draw string to get all the juice out of the pulp.

Dehydrator A dehydrator is used to dry foods at low temperatures (below 47.7°C/118°F) whilst preserving the nutrient content and enzymes of the food. These are expensive, but worth the investment if you are planning to include more raw food in your diet long term. They are perfect for creating "cooked-like" dishes, warming foods or making crackers, chips, breads and wraps. While there are a number of recipes in the book that use a dehydrator, many modern ovens are able to cook at low temperatures (40°C/115°F) and can be used instead (see opposite). For wet mixtures, such as vegetables coated in a marinade or crackers and breads, you will need to line the shelves before starting dehydrating. Most dehydrators come with specially fitted non-stick lining sheets for this purpose. I recommend a dehydrator set at 40°C/115°F for the recipes in this book. Choose one with a built-in timer.

Conventional oven If you do not own a dehydrator, it is still possible to dry out foods, but you need to check the temperature settings of your oven. Set your oven to the lowest setting possible and prop the door open with a wooden spoon, for example. The oven should feel warm, not hot. If it is a fan-assisted oven, there will be more air circulation in the oven, which may speed up dehydration. If it is a conventional oven, you will need to stir or turn over the food every 3–4 hours to ensure it dries evenly. Because a conventional oven may not be as efficient as a dehydrator, you might need to allow more time to dry foods.

Mini grinder Use a clean coffee grinder to process seeds, nuts, herbs and spices in small batches. This is particularly useful for chia and sesame seeds.

Spiralizer This is a simple, inexpensive gadget that creates fine vegetable noodles to make "raw pasta". Although not actually required for any of these recipes, it is a useful gadget if you are planning to include more raw dishes in your diet. It can create a range of different noodle styles, making it ideal for pad thai salads and coleslaws too. Alternatively, you can use the grating or chopping attachment of a food processor, a swivel potato peeler, mandolin or sharp knife.

Mandolin This is not necessary for any of the recipes in the book but is useful for slicing vegetables and fruit thinly.

Sprouter For only a small outlay you can buy sprouters that are very efficient at producing sprouted seeds and beans, but you can also make use of large jam jars covered with a mesh lid or piece of muslin. Alternatively, you can now buy ready-to-eat sprouted seeds and beans.

soaking and sprouting

Soaking nuts and seeds before using them improves their digestibility by helping to reduce the plant's enzyme inhibitors. It also makes them easier to blend in recipes. Simply cover with fresh cold water and leave for the stated time in the recipe (or, for ease, overnight), then rinse and drain thoroughly before using.

Beans, pulses, grains and certain seeds require soaking and sprouting before they can be eaten raw. Kidney beans should never be eaten raw, as they contain a dangerous toxin. (Note, though, that raw dry oats do not need to be soaked or sprouted and can be milled down to be used in raw cake and cookie recipes.) Sprouting not only increases digestibility but also greatly enhances the seeds' nutritional profile. Sprouting is essentially germinating the plant, creating a "living food". This leads to a rapid increase in the vitamin content, as well as making the protein, carbohydrates and fats in the food easier to digest and assimilate. In addition, these living foods are packed with energizing and health-promoting enzymes. Try to include them regularly in your diet to boost your intake of essential nutrients and antioxidants as well as helping to support your digestive system.

soaking times

Seed	Soaking Time	Sprouting Time
Alfalfa	4–6 hours	5 days
Broccoli	4–8 hours	3–4 days
Buckwheat	Overnight	2–3 days
Clover	5–6 hours	5 days
Fenugreek	Overnight	3–5 days

Seed	Soaking Time	Sprouting Time
Kale	4–5 hours	5 days
Mustard	5 hours	5 days
Quinoa	2–3 hours	1–2 days
Radish	Overnight	5 days
Sunflower	4–5 hours	2 days
Bean		
Aduki	Overnight	5–6 days
Chickpeas	Overnight	3–4 days
Lentils	4–8 hours	3–4 days
Mung	Overnight	5 days
Peas	Overnight	3–4 days
Pinto beans	Overnight	3 days
Grain		
Barley	Overnight	5–7 days
Millet	Overnight	2–3 days
Oat groats	6–8 hours	2–3 days
Rye	6–8 hours	5–7 days
Wheat	Overnight	5–7 days
Wild rice	Overnight (min. 9 hours)	3–5 days

green smoothies and raw juices

Raw vegetable juices and blended green smoothies provide plenty of live enzymes, vitamins and minerals in an easily digested form to help nourish and bring energy to the body. Drinking is one of the easiest and quickest ways to get nutrient-rich foods into your diet plus keeping the body hydrated. By blending whole fruits and vegetables, you add water and fibre to help fill you up while cleansing the body, so perfect for helping you to lose weight.

A variety of drinks have been included in the diet plans. Smoothies, nut milks and juices are featured, but feel free to experiment with your own blends. By adding nuts or seeds to a smoothie, you also provide the body with essential proteins to help balance blood sugar levels and stave off hunger pangs.

Vegetable juices and blends of fruit and vegetables are preferred over pure fruit juices since they have a lower glycemic index. Pure fruit juices can upset blood sugar levels which can contribute to fluctuating energy levels, fatigue and potentially sugar cravings. Instead, by focusing more on vegetable blends as well as adding some protein such as nuts and seeds to create a smoothie or shake, you can create a more sustaining drink bursting with nutrients to keep you energized.

Green smoothies and vegetable juices are particularly beneficial as they are not only cleansing but also extremely alkaline – good for balancing acidic bodies that commonly arise due to our stressful lifestyles and poor diets. They are also an excellent way of cramming more greens into your diet. You can mask the slightly bitter flavour by blending in a little fresh fruit. You can always include a pinch of stevia for natural sweetness as well, if needed. It is important through the day that you drink sufficient liquid– your body needs at least six to eight glasses of water each day, but some of this can come from juices, smoothies and raw soups. One of the great things about a raw food diet is that it is naturally very hydrating. Fatigue and cravings can be a sign that your body is dehydrated, so be sure you listen to your body and drink sufficient fluids while on the diet plan.

fermented foods and pickles

Pickling and fermenting foods is a great way of preserving them and creating a wonderful tangy, slightly sour flavour. These foods are a good source of probiotic bacteria (lactobacilli), which support the immune function, digestive health and assimilation of nutrients. They are also packed with vitamins, minerals and enzymes. As they are pre-digested by being fermented, they are usually gentler on the digestive tract and make a useful way of moving to an all raw food diet. Fermented drinks, such as coconut kefir, kombucha and rejuvelac, are equally beneficial and encourage elimination of waste, making them a great addition to a weight-loss programme.

Sauerkraut
This is one of the most common and easy-to-make pickled vegetables. Just put some thinly sliced or grated cabbage into an airtight container with a clamp-down lid and pour over just enough brine solution made using 1 tbsp sea salt to 250ml/9fl oz/1 cup water to cover. Seal the container, then leave the cabbage to ferment. Skim off any skin that forms on the top of the mixture every 1–2 days. Depending on the temperature, it should be ready in around 4 days, but often tastes better after 1– 2 weeks. Once it is fermented, store in the fridge.

Kimchi is a Korean-style method of fermenting cabbage with other vegetables and contains additional spices, such as grated garlic, ginger and chilli powder.

Pickles can be made instantly from either a vinegar or brine solution seasoned with spices or herbs. Any vegetables can be used, but cauliflower, carrot, cucumber, onions, daikon, radish and peppers are all good choices. Simply combine 250ml/9fl oz/1 cup each of cider vinegar and water in a large bowl or jar. Stir in 1 tsp sea salt, a pinch of xylitol or other sweetener, and a range of spices, such as mustard seeds, black peppercorns, coriander seeds, allspice and cinnamon. Next, add a selection of prepared vegetables. Seal and shake to mix, then leave overnight before using.

basic recipes

almond milk

Nut and seed milks are delicious with cereals and added to sauces, soups, smoothies and sweet dishes.

SOAKING TIME: *30 minutes to 2 hours, or overnight if preferable* • **PREPARATION TIME:** *5 minutes* • **STORAGE:** *will keep in the fridge for up to 1–2 days* • **SERVES:** *4*

125g/4½oz/heaped ¾ cup almonds (soaked for 30 minutes–2 hours in 750ml/26fl oz/ 3 cups water) • 3–4 pitted dates

1 Drain the almonds well, retaining the soaking water, and rinse.
2 Place the almonds in a blender with the water and dates and process until smooth. Serve immediately or pour through a nut milk bag or piece of muslin placed over a sieve. Store in the fridge until needed.

Nutritional analysis per serving: *Calories 193kcal • Protein 6.6g • Carbohydrates 2.4g • Fat 17.4g (of which saturates 1.4g)*

VARIATIONS:
Vanilla Add the seeds from 1 vanilla pod or use 2 tsp vanilla extract.
Chocolate Add 2 tbsp raw cacao powder.
Strawberry Add 225g/8oz/1½ cups strawberries and 1 tsp vanilla extract.
Supergreens Add 1 tbsp green superfood powder, e.g. chlorella, barley grass or spirulina, and a little extra sweetener.
Chai Add ½ tsp cinnamon, a pinch each of ground cardamom and nutmeg, ½ tsp vanilla extract.
Sweet Toffee Use 1 tbsp yacon syrup or 6 pitted dates, 2 tbsp mesquite powder and a pinch of cinnamon.
Speedy Nut Butter Milk Use 4½ tsp almond or cashew nut butter and blend with 250ml/9fl oz/1 cup water. Sweeten with a couple of pitted dates, if you like.

basic nut cheese

Raw vegan cheese is made by processing nuts and seeds into a cream-like cheese. While any nut or seed can be used, the most popular include pine nuts, macadamias, cashews, almonds, pecans and sunflower seeds. All raw vegan cheeses are full of protein and calcium for satisfying your appetite as well as providing essential nutrients for weight loss.

SOAKING TIME: *overnight* • **PREPARATION TIME:** *5 minutes* • **STORAGE:** *will keep in the fridge for up to 3 days* • **SERVES:** *4–6*

125g/4½oz/heaped ¾ cup macadamia nuts (soaked overnight, then drained) • 125g/4½oz/heaped ¾ cup cashew nuts (soaked overnight, then drained) • 1 tsp sea salt • 2 tbsp lemon juice • 2 tbsp dried nutritional yeast flakes • 2 tsp onion powder

1 Place the nuts in a food processor and process to form small pieces. Add the remaining ingredients and 185–250ml/6–9fl oz/¾–1 cup water and process until the mixture is creamy and smooth. Serve immediately.
2 Alternatively, for a firmer texture, use a little less water and then spoon the mixture into a muslin-lined colander. Fold the muslin over the cheese and place a weight on the top. Leave to drain for 24 hours to firm up. Transfer to the fridge to harden, then shape into a round.

Nutritional analysis per tablespoon: *Calories 54kcal • Protein 1.3g • Carbohydrates 1.1g • Fat 5g (of which saturates 0.8g)*

VARIATIONS:
Tomato Cheese Blend in 1 chopped tomato, then stir in 4 chopped sun-dried tomatoes.
Sweet Cheese Replace the water with coconut water and add 2 tbsp yacon syrup.
Herb Cheese Add 1 handful herbs, such as basil or rosemary.
Olive Cheese Blend in 1 handful pitted black olives.
Harissa Cheese Replace the macadamia and cashew nuts with 300g/10½oz/scant 2 cups pine nuts, and add 1 dried chipotle pepper, 1 chopped tomato and 1 minced garlic clove.

vegan nut mayonnaise

Use this as a tasty dressing to spread on flaxseed crackers, as a dip, or as a filling for vegetables.

SOAKING TIME: *2 hours* • PREPARATION TIME: *10 minutes* • STORAGE: *will keep in the fridge for up to 4 days*

125g/4½oz/heaped ¾ cup cashew nuts (soaked for 2 hours, then drained) • 2 tbsp cider vinegar • ½ tsp sea salt • 2 tbsp chopped red onion or shallots • 2 tsp yacon syrup or xylitol

1 Place all the ingredients in a blender with 4 tbsp water and blend until smooth and creamy.

Nutritional analysis per tablespoon: *Calories 47kcal • Protein 1.4g • Carbohydrates 2g • Fat 3.8g (of which saturates 0.7g)*

sweet caesar dressing

Creamy, yet low in saturated fat, this delicious dressing is an easy way to dress up any salad dish and will provide plenty of protein to keep energy levels high.

PREPARATION TIME: *5 minutes* • STORAGE: *will keep in the fridge for up to 3–4 days*

60g/2¼oz/heaped ⅓ cup pine nuts • 1 garlic clove • 2 celery stalks • 2 tbsp lemon juice • 2 tbsp cider vinegar • 2 tbsp tamari soy sauce • 1 tbsp white miso • 1 tbsp yacon syrup or xylitol

1 Place all the ingredients in a blender with 125ml/4fl oz/½ cup water and blend until smooth and creamy.

Nutritional analysis per tablespoon: *Calories 21kcal • Protein 0.5g • Carbohydrates 1g • Fat 1.8g (of which saturates 0.1g)*

sun-dried tomato sauce

Serve this low-fat treat with burgers, use as a sauce or blend with some mayonnaise to make a thousand island-style dressing.

PREPARATION TIME: *10 minutes* • **STORAGE:** *will keep in the fridge for up to 3–4 days*

3 ripe plum tomatoes • ¼ red onion, chopped • 60g/2¼oz/heaped ⅓ cup sun-dried tomatoes, chopped • 90g/3¼oz/ ½ cup pitted dates • 1 tsp onion powder • 1 tbsp cider vinegar • 2 tbsp tamari soy sauce

1 Place all the ingredients in a blender and blend until smooth.
2 Add a little water to thin, if needed.

Nutritional analysis per tablespoon: *Calories 15kcal • Protein 0.2g • Carbohydrates 1g • Fat 1.1g (of which saturates 0.1g)*

lemon & herb marinated olives

A useful accompaniment to meals or a healthy snack.

PREPARATION TIME: *15 minutes, plus 2 days to marinate* • **STORAGE:** *will keep in the fridge for up to 1–2 weeks*

½ lemon, thinly sliced • peel of 1 lemon • 2 tbsp lemon juice • 2 shallots, chopped • 1 tbsp chopped rosemary leaves • 1 tbsp chopped oregano • 350g/12oz/heaped 2¾ cups pitted olives • 270ml/9½fl oz/ 1 generous cup extra virgin olive oil

1 Place all the ingredients in a large sterilized glass jar, using just enough oil to cover the olives.
2 Seal the jar and shake to combine. Place in the fridge and leave to marinate for 2 days before using.

Nutritional analysis per tablespoon: *Calories 62kcal • Protein 0.1g • Carbohydrates 0.1g • Fat 6.9g (of which saturates 1g)*

tomato & pepper flaxseed crackers

These low-calorie crackers are the perfect addition to snacks, meals, dips and spreads. Vary the flavours according to taste.

PREPARATION TIME: *15 minutes* • **DEHYDRATING TIME:** *10–11 hours or overnight* • **MAKES:** *20–24 crackers* • **STORAGE:** *keep in an airtight container for up to 1 week*

300g/10½oz/1¾ heaped cups whole flaxseeds • 1 red pepper, halved lengthways, deseeded and chopped • 1 tomato, chopped • 2 sun-dried tomatoes, chopped • 3–4 tbsp lemon juice • ½ tsp sea salt, to taste

1 Place the flaxseeds in a food processor and process until fine. Add the remaining ingredients and blend to form a stiff paste, using enough of 185ml/6fl oz/¾ cup water to form a thick, spreadable dough.
2 Spread the dough into a square or rectangle on a non-stick sheet placed on a baking or dehydrator tray. The dough should be about 5mm/¼in thick. Score lines into the dough to make individual crackers.
3 Put in a dehydrator set at 45°C/115°F for 5–6 hours, then flip over. Dry for a further 5 hours until dry and crispy. Alternatively, place in an oven at 45°C/115°F (or on its lowest setting with the door ajar) and leave overnight. Flip over and bake for a further 4–5 hours until crisp. Break into individual crackers along the score lines.

Nutritional analysis per cracker: *Calories 70kcal • Protein 2.3g • Carbohydrates 4g • Fat 5.4g (of which saturates 0.5g)*

VARIATIONS:
Date or Raisin Crackers To the ground flaxseeds add 125g/4½oz/heaped ⅔ cup pitted dates or 125g/4½oz/1 cup raisins (soaked, then drained), and the juice of 1 orange. Use the date-soaking liquid to form a thick dough.
Berry Crackers Blend 250g/9oz mixed fresh berries and 4 pitted dates with 100g/3½oz/ 1 cup ground flaxseeds. Add 1 tbsp berry antioxidant powder and enough water to form a thick dough.

spiced seeds

These delicious nibbles are the perfect snack to keep you going between meals. A low-fat alternative to potato crisps.

SOAKING TIME: *1 hour* • **PREPARATION TIME:** *10 minutes* • **DEHYDRATION TIME:** *10 hours or overnight* • **STORAGE:** *will keep in an airtight container for up to 3–4 days*

1 tomato • 1 garlic clove • 1 tbsp xylitol or yacon syrup • 1 tsp smoked paprika • 2 tsp tamari soy sauce • 1 tsp sea salt • 2 tbsp olive oil • 250g/9oz/1²/₃ cups mixed pumpkin and sunflower seeds (soaked for 1 hour, then drained)

1 Place all the ingredients except the seeds in a blender and blend to form a sauce.
2 Toss the seeds in the sauce. Spread out the seeds over a non-stick sheet placed on a baking or dehydrator tray. Put in a dehydrator set at 45°C/115°F for 10 hours or overnight. Alternatively, place in an oven at 45°C/115°F (or on its lowest setting with the door ajar) and leave for 8 hours until dry and crisp.

Nutritional analysis per tablespoon: *Calories 43kcal • Protein 1.1g • Carbohydrates 1.7g • Fat 3.6g (of which saturates 0.5g)*

lucuma & cinnamon nuts

Adding lucuma powder creates a sensational caramel-scented coating for nuts, which makes a delicious snack during the day for satisfying those hunger pangs. Cinnamon is a wonderful spice for improving the function of insulin, helping to keep blood sugar levels even and avoiding energy dips and cravings.

SOAKING TIME: *1 hour* • **PREPARATION TIME:** *10 minutes* • **DEHYDRATION TIME:** *8 hours* • **STORAGE:** *will keep in an airtight container for up to 3–4 days*

2 tbsp lucuma powder • 2 tbsp xylitol or yacon syrup • 1 tbsp olive oil • ½ tsp sea salt • 1 tsp cinnamon • 1 tsp vanilla extract • 125g/4½oz/heaped ¾ cup mixed cashew nuts, hazelnuts and almonds (soaked for 1 hour, then drained)

1 Put all the ingredients except the nuts in a bowl and mix to form a paste.
2 Toss the nuts in the paste. Spread on a non-stick sheet placed on a baking or dehydrator tray. Put in a dehydrator set at 45°C/115°F for 8 hours or overnight. Alternatively, place in an oven at 45°C/115°F (or on its lowest setting with the door ajar) and leave until dry (around 4 hours).

Nutritional analysis per tablespoon: *Calories 70kcal • Protein 2.1g • Carbohydrates 4.6g • Fat 5.1g (of which saturates 0.8g)*

wraps, tortillas & corn chips

Use the following recipe and variation for healthy raw corn wraps or tortillas. The recipe can also be made into chips, which are a perfect accompaniment to soups and dips.

SOAKING TIME: *30 minutes* • **PREPARATION TIME:** *15 minutes* • **DEHYDRATION TIME:** *8–10 hours (wraps/tortillas) or 6–8 hours (corn chips)* • **MAKES:** *6 wraps* • **STORAGE:** *will keep for up to 2 days*

310g/11oz/1½ cups sweetcorn, scraped off the cob or frozen • ¼ red onion • 40g/1½oz/ heaped ⅓ cup ground flaxseeds (soaked for 30 minutes, then drained) • 1 tbsp lime juice • ½ tsp sea salt • 3 tbsp olive oil • pinch each cayenne pepper, chilli powder and cumin

1 Place the corn and onion in a food processor and process to form a purée. Add the remaining ingredients and process to form a smooth batter.
2 To make wraps or tortillas, spread the batter into 6 circles on non-stick sheets placed on three baking or dehydrator trays. Put in a dehydrator set at 45°C/115°F, or place in an oven at 45°C/115°F (or on its lowest setting with the door ajar), for 4–6 hours. Flip over when the top is dry. Continue drying for another 4 hours until the wrap/tortillla is dry but still pliable.
3 To make chips, spread the batter over the non-stick sheets to form a rectangle and score the mixture into little squares. Dehydrate as above, for about 6–8 hours, until crisp. Break into squares.

Nutritional analysis per wrap: *Calories 161kcal • Protein 3g • Carbohydrates 10.8g • Fat 12g (of which saturates 1.2g)*

VARIATION:
Courgette Wraps Instead of sweetcorn, onion and spices, use 2 grated courgettes, 100g/3½oz/1 cup ground flaxseeds, plus a few fresh or dried herbs and 125ml/4fl oz/ ½ cup water to form a thick batter.

courgette almond bread

A delicious raw flatbread recipe. Instead of almonds you could use the dried almond pulp left over from making Almond Milk (see page 24). You could also pulse in some herbs or crushed garlic for additional flavour. For a sweet option, replace the courgette with an apple or pear.

PREPARATION TIME: *15 minutes* • **DEHYDRATING TIME:** *11–18 hours* • **MAKES:** *16 slices* • **STORAGE:** *will keep for up to 2–3 days*

400g/14oz/heaped 2½ cups almonds • 115g/4oz/heaped ⅔ cup whole flaxseeds • 1 tsp sea salt • 1 courgette, chopped • 2 tbsp olive oil • 1 tbsp dried nutritional yeast flakes (optional) • freshly ground black pepper

1 Place the almonds and flaxseeds in a food processor and process until fine. Place in a bowl with the salt.
2 Put the remaining ingredients in the food processor with 2 tbsp water and blend to form a purée. Mix into the dry ingredients to form a dough, adding a little more water if the dough is too dry.
3 Form into a thin rectangular loaf about 2.5cm/1in thick on a non-stick sheet placed on a baking or deydrator tray. Mark into slices with a knife and put in a dehydrator set at 45°C/115°F for 10 hours, or place in an oven at 45°C/115°F (or on its lowest setting with the door ajar) for 10–12 hours. Flip over and dehydrate for a further 1–4 hours, depending on how dry you want the bread.

Nutritional analysis per slice: *Calories 213kcal • Protein 7.2g • Carbohydrates 4.2g • Fat 18.9g (of which saturates 1.7g)*

pizza base

This is equally delicious as a tart base for savoury quiches or tarts. Simply press into tart tins and dehydrate as below.

PREPARATION TIME: *30 minutes* • **DEHYDRATING TIME:** *4–6 hours* • **SERVES:** *6* • **STORAGE:** *will keep for up to 2–3 days*

125g/4½oz/1 cup sunflower seeds • 100g/3½oz/1 cup ground flaxseeds • 2 carrots, chopped • ½ tsp sea salt or garlic salt • 1 tbsp dried oregano • 1 tbsp olive oil

1 Place the sunflower seeds in a food processor and process to form a fine flour. Place in a bowl with the flaxseeds.
2 Place the remaining ingredients and 125ml/4fl oz/½ cup water in the food processor and process until smooth. Pour the purée into the seeds and mix well to form a stiff dough. Allow to stand for 15 minutes before using.
3 Spread the dough into a thin circle on a non-stick sheet placed on a baking or dehydrator tray. Put in a dehydrator set at 45°C/115°F, or place in an oven at 45°C/115°F (or on its lowest setting with the door ajar), for 4–6 hours to dry before topping.

Nutritional analysis per serving: *Calories 238kcal • Protein 6.6g • Carbohydrates 9.6g • Fats 19.6g (of which saturates 1.8g)*

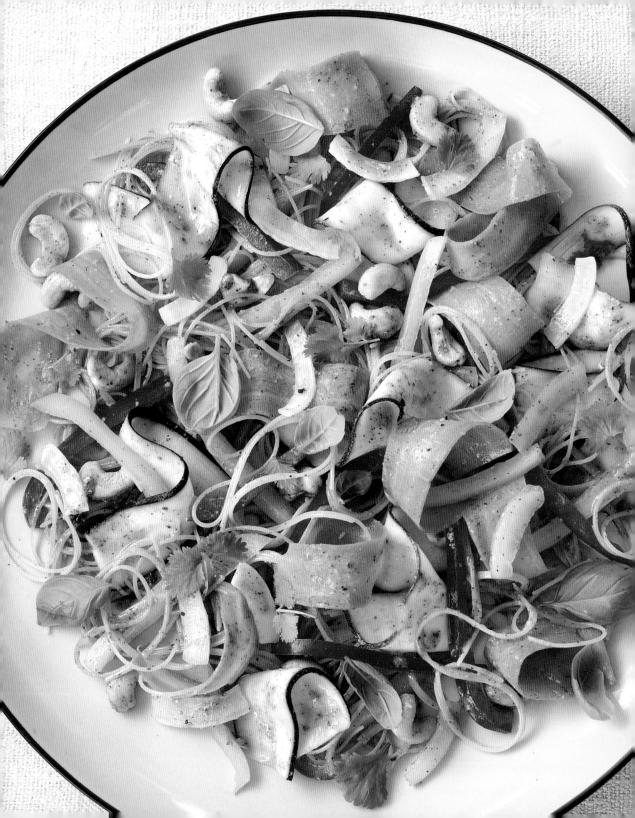

CHAPTER 1

The Raw Food Weekend Blitz Diet

Do you look in the mirror and wonder what has happened to your body and energy levels? Are you fed up with trying to lose weight and getting nowhere, or do you just wake up tired and lethargic and struggle to get through the day? If so, the Weekend Blitz Diet is the perfect kick-start to a new you. Within just one weekend of eating raw food, you will feel younger and slimmer. You will feel more in control of your eating and will have started to transform your body by giving it the nutrients it needs to be healthier and leaner.

In this chapter you will find some weekend menus. Enjoy a range of cleansing, energizing juices and smoothies, raw muesli, creamy soup, salads, sushi, raw burgers and a delicious raw fruit bar. By the end of the weekend, you'll feel lighter and slimmer and re-energized.

< pad thai (page 48)

the raw food weekend programme

To maximize the benefits of your raw weekend, it is important that you plan to succeed, so take time to prepare for your weekend carefully. Choose a weekend free of commitments or too much stress.

Read through the menu plan and recipes and ensure you have everything you need. Most of the recipes can be prepared in advance. Flaxseed crackers, for example, require overnight drying, so start these a couple of days earlier. You can also make the burgers, the raw bar and muesli in advance. Other recipes, such as nut milks, soup and Spiced Plums with Ginger Cream, can be made the day before if you like. While some recipes suggest using a dehydrator, this is not necessary, and the recipes work equally well in a conventional oven set on its lowest setting (see text on dehydrators, page 18).

Preparation A week before you start the weekend programme, gradually build up your intake of raw food. Try to have one meal a day that is all raw – for example, a large mixed salad with sprouted seeds for lunch or a raw breakfast. At the same time, begin to cut back on processed foods and stimulants, including alcohol, caffeine, sugary foods and drinks and ready meals.

The weekend programme begins on Friday evening with a green juice and raw vegetable meal. During the day on the Friday, avoid all meat and dairy foods and eat lightly, focusing on vegetables, fruit, nuts and seeds, plus protein such as eggs or fish.

For each day of the programme ensure you drink at least 6 glasses (1.5l/52fl oz/ 6 cups) plain, filtered water and start each day with a glass of warm water and lemon juice to encourage cleansing. You can also drink herbal teas and green tea throughout the day for a warming drink. A juice or smoothie is included daily because these are incredibly nourishing and will simultaneously help to cleanse the body.

the raw food weekend blitz plan

Friday evening

Green Piña Colada Shake (**page 38**),
Pad Thai (**page 48**), herbal tea

Saturday

On waking Large glass of warm water
with juice of ½ lemon

Breakfast Lemon Wheatgrass Shot
(**page 38**), Spiced Plums with Ginger
Cream (**page 40**)

Lunch Creamy Corn Chowder with
Coriander (**page 45**)

Snack Carrot & Lemon Spice Juice
(**page 39**), Flaxseed Crackers (**page 28**)

Dinner Nori Rolls with Sushi "Rice" &
Sesame Lemon Dipping Sauce
(**page 51**), Asian Sea Greens Salad
(**page 56**)

Sunday

On waking Large glass of warm water
with juice of ½ lemon

Breakfast Energy Bomb (**page 39**),
Coconut, Flax & Cinnamon Muesli
(**page 43**) with Almond Milk (**page 24**)

Lunch Avocado, Citrus & Spiced Seed
Salad with Olive Vinaigrette (**page 46**),
Flaxseed Crackers (**page 28**)

Snack Black Forest Cherry Bar (**page 59**),
Spiced Seeds (**page 29**)

Dinner Sunflower Seed Burgers with
Sweet Chilli Tomato Sauce (**page 52**),
Apple, Carrot & Fennel Coleslaw
(**page 55**)

The menu includes many leafy greens, which are alkalizing, nutrient rich and release their natural sugars slowly, thereby helping to stabilize blood sugar levels while keeping energy levels high. While it is recommended that you follow the suggested menu plan, you can swap meal options around according to taste.

A snack suggestion is included, but it is important to listen to your true appetite: eat only when hungry and chew food thoroughly. Try to eat early in the evening – ideally by 7pm – to enable your body to digest food thoroughly before bedtime, helping avoid bloating, a heavy stomach, digestive upsets and disturbed sleep.

breakfasts

lemon wheatgrass shot

An invigorating, cleansing juice that is perfect to kick-start your weight-loss plan. This refreshing green cocktail will speed up the elimination of toxins to help blast stubborn fat.

PREPARATION TIME: *10 minutes* ● **STORAGE:** *best drunk immediately, but will keep in the fridge for 24 hours* ● **SERVES:** *1*

---

2 apples ● **2 tbsp wheatgrass juice or 1 handful wheatgrass** ● **2 celery sticks** ● **1 lemon**

1 Juice all the ingredients and blend well.

HEALTH BENEFITS
*Wheatgrass is very rich in health-boosting nutrients, including energizing **chlorophyll**. It is also a great source of **vitamins B, C and E and carotene**, which are very effective in **destroying free radicals**. Packed with **amino acids**, it can also aid **cell regeneration and growth**.*

Nutritional analysis per serving: *Calories 80kcal* ● *Protein 1.2g* ● *Carbohydrates 16.8g* ● *Fat 0.4g (of which saturates 0.1g)*

green piña colada shake

A creamy-tasting tropical smoothie, rich in digestive enzymes and cleansing ingredients to keep you trim and vibrant.

PREPARATION TIME: *10 minutes + 4 hours freezing time* ● **STORAGE:** *best drunk immediately* ● **SERVES:** *2*

---

1 banana, sliced ● **1 large handful spinach leaves** ● **½ cucumber, peeled and chopped** ● **½ pineapple, chopped** ● **2 tbsp unsweetened, dried, shredded coconut flakes** ● **500ml/17fl oz/2 cups coconut water**

1 Put the banana in a lidded container and freeze for 4 hours or overnight.
2 Place all the ingredients in a blender and blend until smooth.

HEALTH BENEFITS
*Pineapple contains the digestive enzyme **bromelain**, which helps **break down protein, reduce inflammation and promote digestion**.*

Nutritional analysis per serving: *Calories 158kcal* ● *Protein 1.7g* ● *Carbohydrates 27.8g* ● *Fat 3.8g (of which saturates 0.1g)*

energy bomb

If you're missing your caffeine fix, try this energizing juice. Green tea is a well-known fat burner, helping to speed up weight loss. If you can't find matcha tea powder, buy loose green tea leaves and grind to a powder in a coffee grinder. Alternatively, cover a green tea bag with a little hot water and allow it to steep for 10 minutes, then add the liquid to the juice.

PREPARATION TIME: *10 minutes* ● **STORAGE:** *best drunk immediately, but will keep in the fridge for 24 hours* ● **SERVES:** 2

1 large cucumber ● 2 pears, peeled ● 1 lemon, peeled ● 2 tsp matcha green tea powder ● ½ tsp green superfood powder

1 Pass the cucumber, pears and lemon through a juicer.
2 Pour into a blender and blend in the powders to serve.

HEALTH BENEFITS
*Green tea is packed full with health-promoting **antioxidants**, including flavonoids, tannins and catechins. It is a great **slimming aid**, shown to **stimulate metabolism and fat burning**.*

Nutritional analysis per serving: *Calories 78kcal ● Protein 1.7g ● Carbohydrates 16.5g ● Fat 0.4g (of which saturates 0g)*

carrot & lemon spice juice

Refreshing and light, this juice is a powerful detoxifying drink to have at breakfast or as a snack. It is bursting with antioxidants to support immune health, while the flaxseeds provide additional fibre to cleanse the body, making you feel lighter and fresher.

PREPARATION TIME: *10 minutes* ● **STORAGE:** *best drunk immediately, but will keep in the fridge for 1 day* ● **SERVES:** 2

4 apples, peeled ● 3 lemons, peeled ● 2 carrots, peeled ● 1 tbsp ground flaxseeds ● ½ tsp cayenne pepper, to taste

1 Pass the apples, lemons and carrots through a juicer.
2 Place in a blender with the flaxseeds and cayenne and blend until smooth.

HEALTH BENEFITS
*A fiery spice, cayenne pepper is a **circulatory stimulant**, helping to **increase blood supply** to all parts of the body, **improve metabolism** and **aid removal of waste** from the body. A fantastic weight-loss and detox aid.*

Nutritional analysis per serving: *Calories 129kcal ● Protein 2.5g ● Carbohydrates 21.5g ● Fat 3.8g (of which saturates 0.1g)*

spiced plums with ginger cream   >

Full of warming spices, this fruit dish is perfect for colder days. The ginger cream is packed with protein and healthy fats to help avoid hunger pangs and energy dips mid-morning.

PREPARATION TIME: *15 minutes, plus 1 hour marinating time* • **STORAGE:** *will keep in the fridge for up to 3 days* • **SERVES:** *4*

8 plums, halved and pitted • 500ml/17fl oz/2 cups red grape or pomegranate juice • 4 star anise • 1 cinnamon stick • 4 tbsp chia seeds

GINGER CREAM: 125g/4½oz/heaped ¾ cup cashew nuts • 1 tsp grated root ginger • 1 tbsp xylitol or yacon syrup • ½ tsp cinnamon • ½ tsp vanilla extract • 2 nectarines, peeled, halved, pitted and sliced

1 Place the plums, juice, star anise and cinnamon stick in a saucepan. Warm through, then turn off the heat and allow to stand for 1 hour. Remove the fruit using a slotted spoon. Strain the juice and reserve.
2 Mix together the juice and the chia seeds in a bowl and leave for 20 minutes to thicken, stirring occasionally. Place in a blender and blend to form a thick, smooth sauce. Add the fruit.
3 To make the cream, place all the ingredients in a blender with 125ml/4fl oz/½ cup water and blend until very smooth.
4 Spoon the fruit and sauce into bowls and top with the cream.

HEALTH BENEFITS
*A well-known medicinal spice, ginger **boosts the circulation** and helps the body to **detoxify**. Good news for slimmers, too, is it may help **speed up metabolism and calorie burning**. A great digestive aid, it also alleviates complaints such as **indigestion** and **nausea**. The powerful **gingerols** possess anti-inflammatory properties known to help **reduce pain and inflammation** and to **alleviate asthma**.*

Nutritional analysis per serving: *Calories 364kcal • Protein 10.2g • Carbohydrates 40g • Fat 19.8g (of which saturates 3g)*

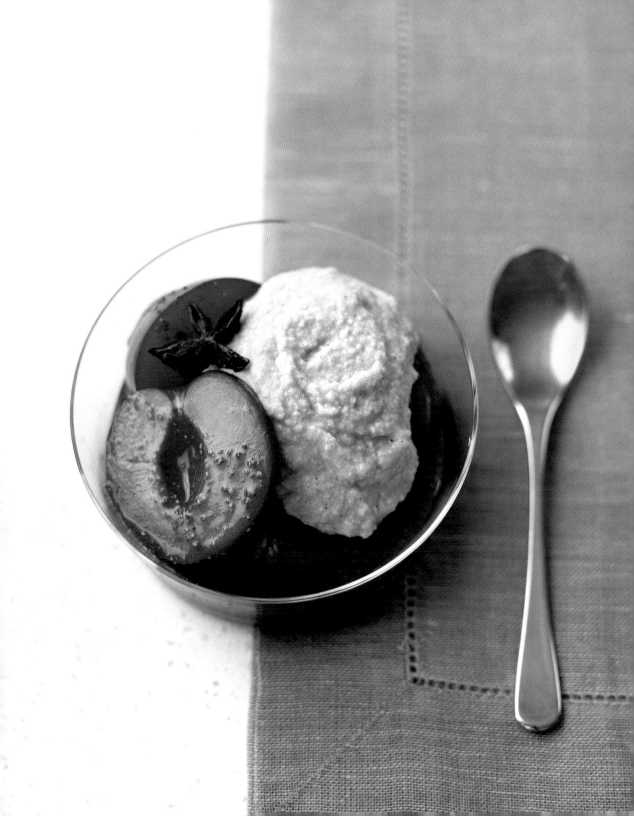

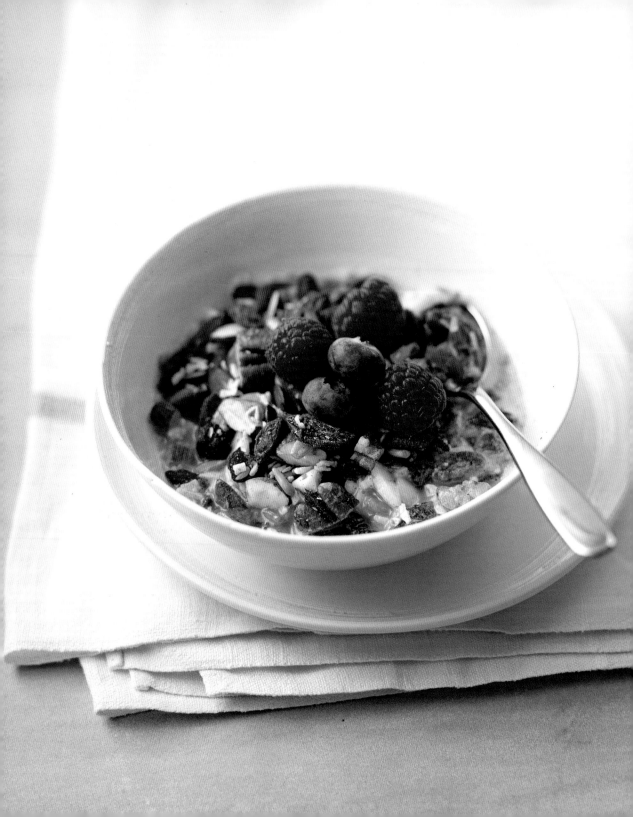

< coconut, flax & cinnamon muesli

Instead of resorting to sugary cereals, try this protein-packed nut and seed muesli. Adding a little cinnamon is a great way to help stabilize blood sugar, allowing you to resist the temptation to snack on unhealthy foods mid-morning. A speedy, nutrient-dense start to the day.

PREPARATION TIME: *10 minutes* • **STORAGE:** *will keep in an airtight container for up to 1 month* • **SERVES:** *6*

55g/2oz/scant 1 cup unsweetened, dried, shredded coconut flakes • 1 tsp cinnamon • 40g/1½oz/heaped ⅓ cup pecans, chopped • 35g/1¼oz/⅓ cup cracked or ground flaxseeds • 4 tbsp pumpkin seeds • 4 tbsp sunflower seeds • 60g/2¼oz/heaped ⅓ cup almonds, roughly chopped • 2 tbsp sesame seeds • 2 tbsp shelled hemp seeds • 55g/2oz/scant ½ cup goji berries • 55g/2oz/½ cup mixed dried berries • 1 recipe quantity Almond Milk (see page 24), to serve • blueberries and raspberries, to serve

1 Place all the ingredients in a bowl and mix well.
2 Spoon into bowls and top with fresh fruit and creamy almond milk to serve.

HEALTH BENEFITS
*Flaxseeds are rich in essential **omega-3 fatty acids**, known to **aid metabolism** and support **weight loss**. They are also packed with **fibre** and **lignans**, which the body converts into hormone-like substances to help **rebalance hormone levels**. Ground flaxseeds are more easily absorbed than whole seeds, making them beneficial for cleansing the body.*

Nutritional analysis per serving (without nut milk or fresh berries): *Calories 352kcal • Protein 10.7g • Carbohydrates 17.7g • Fat 26.6g (of which saturates 2.9g)*

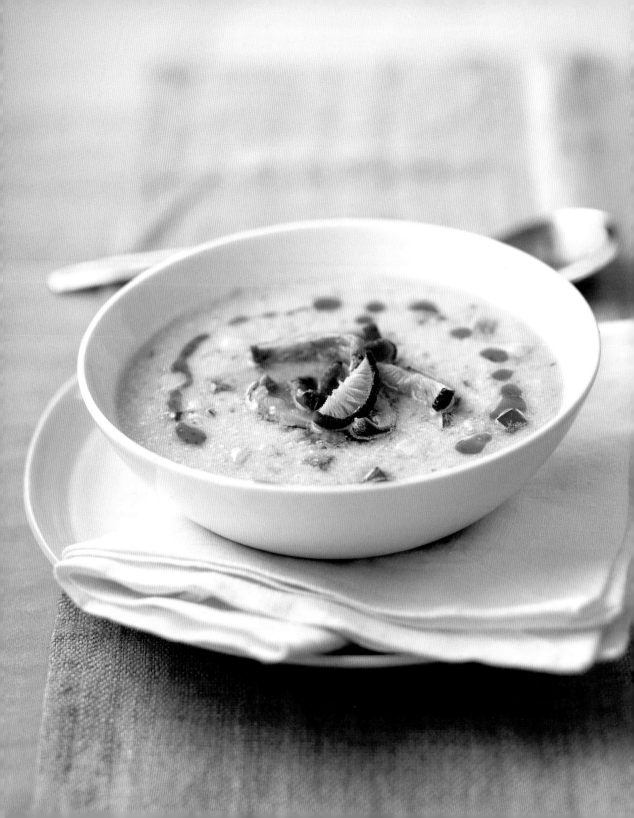

lunches

< creamy corn chowder with coriander

A creamy-tasting, hearty soup, perfect for a snack or light lunch. Adding a few cashew nuts and spices enhances the richness of the dish.

SOAKING TIME: *2 hours* ● **PREPARATION TIME:** *20 minutes* ● **STORAGE:** *the chowder will keep in the fridge for up to 3 days. The coriander oil will keep in the fridge for up to 1 week* ● **SERVES:** *4*

30g/1oz/1 cup coriander leaves • 4 tbsp extra virgin olive oil or flaxseed oil • pinch sea salt • 60g/2¼oz/heaped ⅓ cup cashew nuts (soaked for 2 hours, then drained) • 500ml/ 17fl oz/ 2 cups coconut water or water • 1 tomato, chopped • 1 garlic clove, minced • 1 tbsp white miso paste • 1 tbsp tamari • ½ red chilli, deseeded and chopped • 325g/11½ oz/scant 2¼ cups frozen sweetcorn kernels, thawed • ½ red pepper, deseeded and diced • 1 handful own dehydrated mushroom slices, or 15g/½oz dried shiitake mushrooms, soaked in warm water for 15 minutes, then drained • freshly ground black pepper

1 To make the coriander oil, place the coriander leaves in a blender with the oil and salt and blend until smooth. Sieve. Store in a bottle in the fridge until needed.
2 Place the cashew nuts and coconut water in a blender and blend until smooth. Add the tomato, garlic, miso, tamari, chilli and three-quarters of the corn kernels. Blend until smooth and creamy. Season with pepper to taste and stir in the remaining corn and the red pepper.
3 Spoon the soup into bowls and drizzle over a little coriander oil. Scatter over the mushrooms. Warm through in a dehydrator or cool oven for 30 minutes, if you like.

HEALTH BENEFITS
*Fresh coriander provides health-boosting **antioxidants: beta-carotene, vitamin C** and **flavonoids**.*

Nutritional analysis per serving: Calories 331kcal • Protein 6.5g • Carbohydrates 21.6g • Fat 24g (of which saturates 3.8g)

avocado, citrus & spiced seed salad with olive vinaigrette >

This easy-to-assemble salad is rich in protein, healthy fats and nutrients to keep you feeling energized throughout the day. Add the spiced seeds for texture. Instead of oranges, try pink grapefruit, if you like.

PREPARATION TIME: *15 minutes* ● **STORAGE:** *best eaten on the same day* ● **SERVES:** *4*

225g/8oz mixed salad leaves, such as watercress, rocket and romaine lettuce ● 2 oranges ● 1 red onion, diced ● 2 avocados, halved, pitted and sliced ● 60g/2oz sprouted seeds, e.g. mung beans, alfalfa, broccoli sprouts (optional) ● 1 tbsp Spiced Seeds (see page 29)

OLIVE VINAIGRETTE: 2 tbsp pitted black olives, finely chopped ● 2 tbsp cider vinegar ● 4 tbsp flaxseed oil or extra virgin olive oil ● pinch of sea salt ● freshly ground black pepper

1 Place the mixed salad leaves on a large platter.
2 Separate the oranges into segments, then remove the membranes. Put in a bowl, reserving any juice in a jug.
3 Add the onion, avocados and seeds (including sprouted seeds, if using) to the oranges. Spoon the mixture over the salad leaves.
4 Add the vinaigrette ingredients to the orange juice and mix well. Season with salt and pepper to taste. Pour over the salad and serve immediately.

HEALTH BENEFITS
Sprouted seeds *are a valuable ingredient in any raw food diet. Not only are they* ***nutritional*** ***powerhouses*** *but they are also packed with* ***enzymes*** *to help your body* ***process and digest food*** *efficiently. These living foods are also great* ***cleansers****: being rich in* ***chlorophyll****, they aid the* ***elimination of toxins*** *while keeping the body alkaline and energized.*

Nutritional analysis per serving: *Calories 302kcal ● Protein 4.3g ● Carbohydrates 7.7g ● Fat 28.1g (of which saturates 4.7g)*

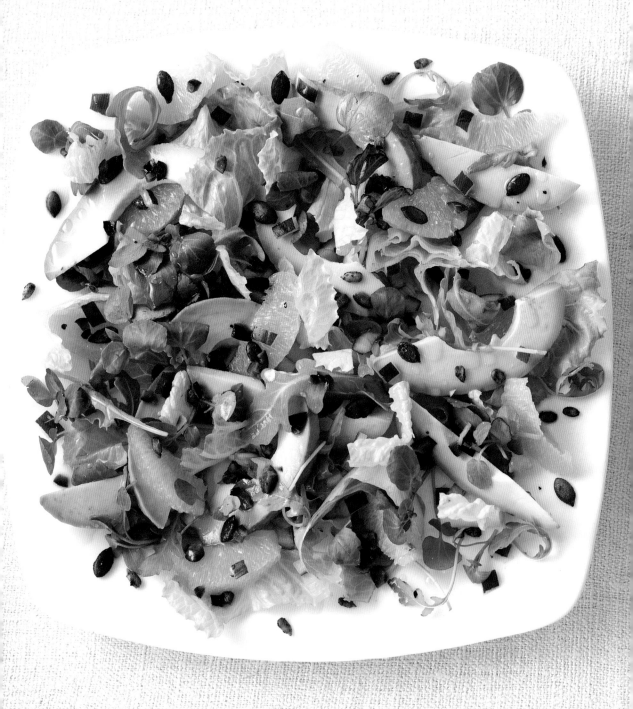

dinners

pad thai >

Creamy, yet light and nourishing, this is the perfect start to your raw weekend. You can prepare this dish in advance, if you want, but toss in the dressing only just before serving. Adding kelp noodles provides additional texture and minerals, which will support metabolism.

SOAKING TIME: *15 minutes* • **PREPARATION TIME:** *15 minutes* • **STORAGE:** *will keep in the fridge for up to 2 days* • **SERVES:** *2*

2 carrots, peeled, spiralized (see page 19) or julienned • 1 courgette, spiralized or julienned • ½ red pepper, deseeded and thinly sliced • ½ yellow pepper, deseeded and thinly sliced • 1 large handful kelp noodles (soaked for 15 minutes, then drained) • 30g/1oz/½ cup unsweetened, dried, shredded coconut flakes • 3 tbsp cashew nuts • handful of mung beans (optional) • 1 small handful Thai basil leaves • 1 small handful coriander leaves (optional)

NUT DRESSING: 3 tbsp almond butter • 1 tbsp lemon juice • 1 tsp xylitol or yacon syrup • 2 tbsp tamari soy sauce • 2 tbsp melted coconut butter (see page 17) • 1 tsp ground cumin • pinch chilli powder or flakes

1 To make the nut dressing, place all the ingredients in a blender and blend to create a thick sauce, adding as much as you need of 80ml/2½fl oz/⅓ cup water.

2 Place all the salad ingredients and noodles in a large bowl and stir in the dressing.

HEALTH BENEFITS
*Almond butter is a fantastic, **protein-packed** spread, rich in **vitamin E, fibre and antioxidants**. It is a great source of healthy **monounsaturated fats**, plus the minerals **magnesium, potassium, manganese and copper**. Almonds can **lower LDL cholesterol** and **stabilize blood sugar levels**.*

Nutritional analysis per serving: *Calories 469kcal • Protein 11.2g • Carbohydrates 18.8g • Fat 40.3g (of which saturates 15.9g)*

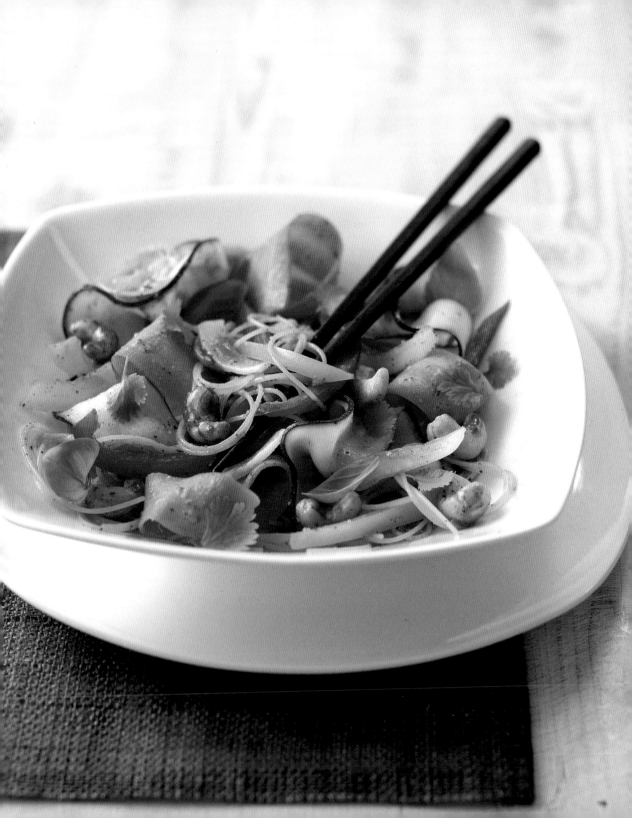

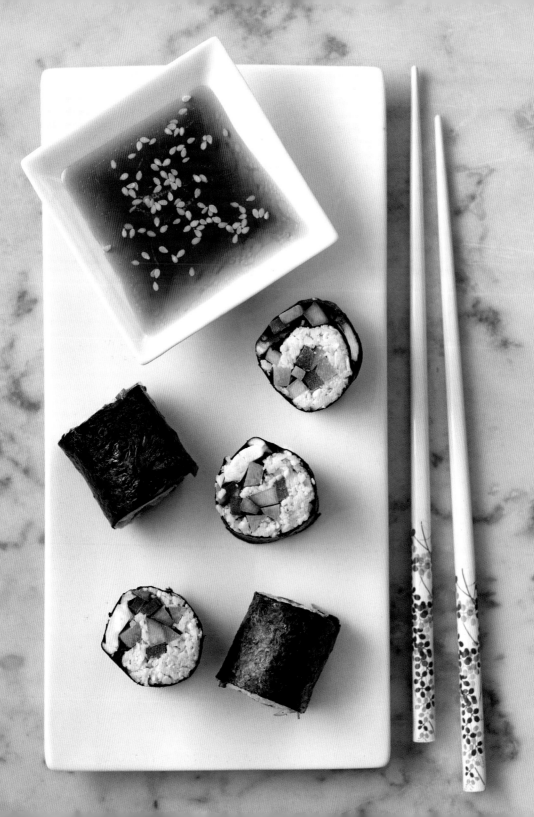

< nori rolls with sushi "rice" & sesame lemon dipping sauce

Sushi is a wonderful treat, and this raw version is simple and easy to prepare. For the filling, use a range of vegetable strips according to taste. For a speedy option, replace the "rice" with one of the pâtés or dips in this book.

PREPARATION TIME: *20 minutes* • **STORAGE:** *will keep in the fridge for up to 1 day* • **SERVES:** *4*

1 recipe quantity cauliflower or parsnip "rice" (see page 90) • 4 nori sheets • 1 red pepper, halved lengthways, deseeded and thinly sliced • ¼ cucumber, julienned • 1 carrot, julienned • 6 shiitake mushrooms, thinly sliced

SESAME LEMON DIPPING SAUCE: 125ml/4fl oz/½ cup rice vinegar • 4 tbsp yacon syrup or xylitol • 1 tbsp tamari soy sauce • ½ tsp sesame oil • finely grated zest of ½ lemon • sprinkling of sesame seeds

1 To make the dipping sauce, whisk together the rice vinegar, yacon syrup, tamari, sesame oil and lemon zest in a bowl. Stir in the sesame seeds.
2 Make the cauliflower or parsnip "rice", adding a little oil to help it stick, if needed.
3 Place a nori sheet shiny side down on a rolling mat. Spread an even layer of the rice across the sheet on the bottom third closest to you. Press down firmly. Place a line of pepper, cucumber and carrot on top, then add some shiitake slices. Dampen the edges of the nori sheet with a little water.
4 Roll up tightly using the mat to help. Repeat with the remaining nori sheets and vegetables. Cut into slices with a serrated knife. Serve with the dipping sauce.

HEALTH BENEFITS
*Shiitake mushrooms contain the phytochemical **lentinan**, which helps **lower cholesterol**, stimulate the **immune system** and **protect against cancers**. It also promotes the production of **interferon**, which has potent **anti-viral** and **anti-bacterial** properties, enhancing overall **immune health**.*

Nutritional analysis per serving: *Calories 160kcal • Protein 5.8g • Carbohydrates 20.3g • Fat 8.1g (of which saturates 0.9g)*

sunflower seed burgers with sweet chilli tomato sauce >

Meaty-style burgers combining rich-tasting Portobello mushroom and nutty-flavoured sunflower seeds. Serve with mixed salad leaves. These burgers are also great as snacks when you are out and about, or as part of a packed lunch.

PREPARATION TIME: *20 minutes* • **DEHYDRATION TIME:** *8–10 hours or overnight* • **STORAGE:** *will keep in the fridge for up to 3 days* • **SERVES:** *4*

40g/1½oz/heaped ⅓ cup ground flaxseeds • 55g/2oz/scant ½ cup sunflower seeds
• 1 tbsp chopped parsley • 1 tbsp flaxseed oil or olive oil • 2 tbsp tamari soy sauce
• 1 garlic clove, minced • 2 tbsp nutritional yeast flakes • ¼ tsp sea salt • ½ tsp Dijon mustard • 1 Portobello mushroom, cut into chunks • salad leaves, to serve

SWEET CHILLI TOMATO SAUCE: ½ recipe quantity Sun-Dried Tomato Sauce (see page 27)
• 1 dried red chilli, rehydrated, deseeded and chopped

1 To make the sauce, blend the tomato sauce and chilli in a blender until fairly smooth.
2 Place all the burger ingredients except the mushroom in a food processor and process until well combined. Add the mushroom and pulse gently until chunky.
3 Shape the mixture into 4 small burgers on a non-stick sheet placed on a baking or dehydrator tray. Put in a dehydrator set at 45°C/115°F for 8–10 hours, turning them over as they dry. Alternatively, place in an oven at 45°C/115°F (or on its lowest setting with the door ajar) overnight. Serve with the sweet chilli tomato sauce and salad.

HEALTH BENEFITS
*Sunflower seeds are little nuggets of goodness, bursting with energizing nutrients, including **magnesium**, **zinc** and **B vitamins**. They are also packed full of **vitamin E**, an antioxidant that helps to keep your body **youthful** and **glowing**.*

Nutritional analysis per serving: *Calories 258kcal • Protein 9.5g • Carbohydrates 13.4g • Fat 19.2g (of which saturates 2g)*

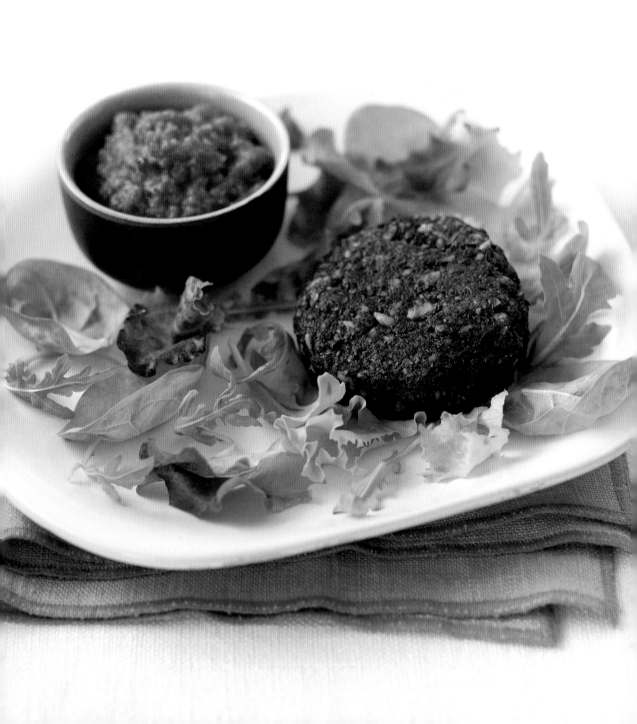

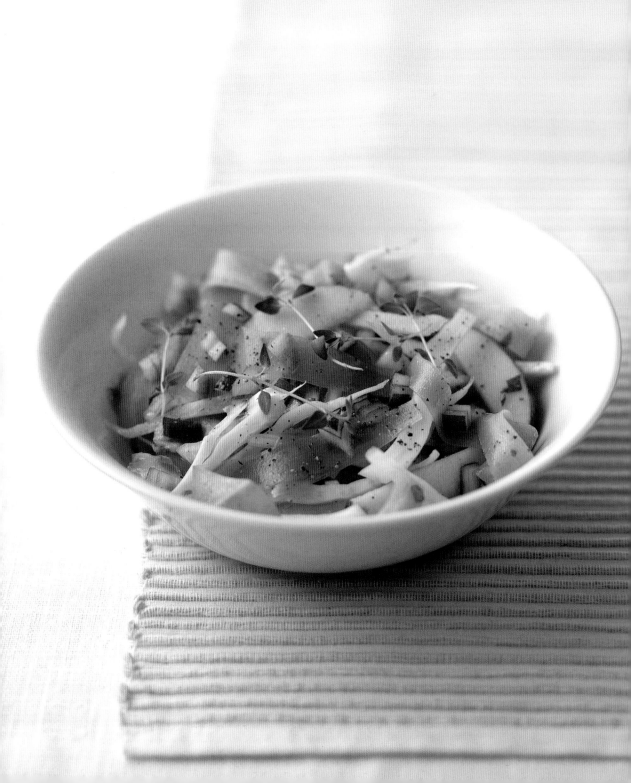

side dishes

< apple, carrot & fennel coleslaw

A light lemon dressing coats this wonderfully refreshing salad, which is perfect on its own or as an accompaniment to a main dish. Fennel and apple are a great weight-loss combination: fennel contains essential oils, such as anethole, which is mildly diuretic, while apples are a powerful cleansing and detoxing food.

PREPARATION TIME: *20 minutes* • **STORAGE:** *will keep in the fridge for up to 2 days* • **SERVES:** *4*

---

1 fennel bulb, julienned • 2 apples, cored and julienned • 2 carrots, peeled and julienned • 1 small red onion, finely chopped • 2 tsp chopped thyme, plus young thyme leaves, to scatter

DRESSING: 2 tbsp lemon juice • 1 tsp finely grated lemon zest • 2 tsp yacon syrup • 4 tbsp hemp oil or flaxseed oil • 1 handful mint leaves, chopped • freshly ground black pepper

1 Place the fennel, apples and carrots in a large bowl with the onion and thyme.
2 Mix together all the dressing ingredients in a bowl.
3 Pour over the salad and toss well just before serving. Season with pepper and scatter with the thyme leaves.

HEALTH BENEFITS
*Fennel is a well-known **digestive aid** and a great source of **potassium** and **fibre**, helping to **eliminate toxins** and **reduce fluid retention**. It also improves **fat digestion** by stimulating the gall bladder and increasing the flow of bile, which **breaks down fat** and **aids its removal**. Rich in **phytoestrogens**, it can help **balance hormone levels**, too.*

Nutritional analysis per serving: *Calories 172kcal • Protein 0.8g • Carbohydrates 8.9g • Fat 15.2g (of which saturates 2.2g)*

asian sea greens salad >

This combination of sea vegetables and salad leaves tossed in an oriental-inspired dressing creates a wonderfully light and refreshing side dish. Use a selection of sea vegetables such as dulse, wakame and sea lettuce for this dish.

SOAKING TIME: *15 minutes* • **PREPARATION TIME:** *10 minutes* • **STORAGE:** *the salad will keep in the fridge for up to 2 days. The dressing will keep in the fridge for up to 1 week* • **SERVES:** *4*

25g/1oz/1 cup mixed sea vegetables (soaked for 15 minutes, then drained) • 1 large handful watercress • 1 large handful rocket leaves • 4 radishes, finely sliced • ½ cucumber, cut into long strips lengthways

DRESSING: 1 tbsp tamari soy sauce • 1 tbsp mirin • 1 tbsp rice vinegar • 1 tsp sesame oil • 2 tsp flaxseed oil

1 Combine all the salad ingredients in a large bowl.
2 Mix together all the dressing ingredients in a bowl.
3 Pour over the salad, toss well and serve.

HEALTH BENEFITS
*Sea vegetables are rich in **minerals**, particularly **iodine** needed for the optimal functioning of the thyroid gland, which is important for **metabolism** and enabling **weight loss**. They also contain **lignans**, which can help **detoxify** the body and may provide protection against certain **cancers**.*

Nutritional analysis per serving: *Calories 53kcal • Protein 3.2g • Carbohydrates 1.3g • Fat 3.8g (of which saturates 0.6g)*

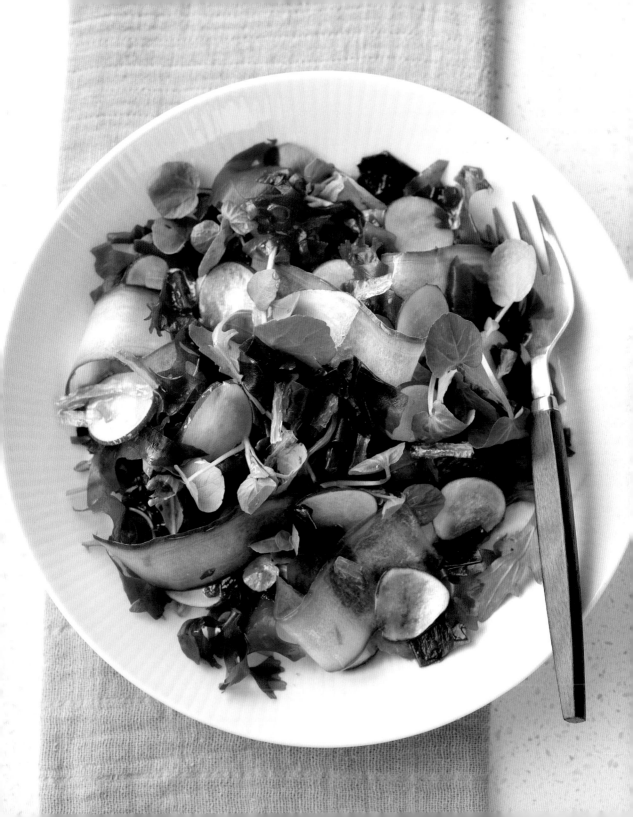

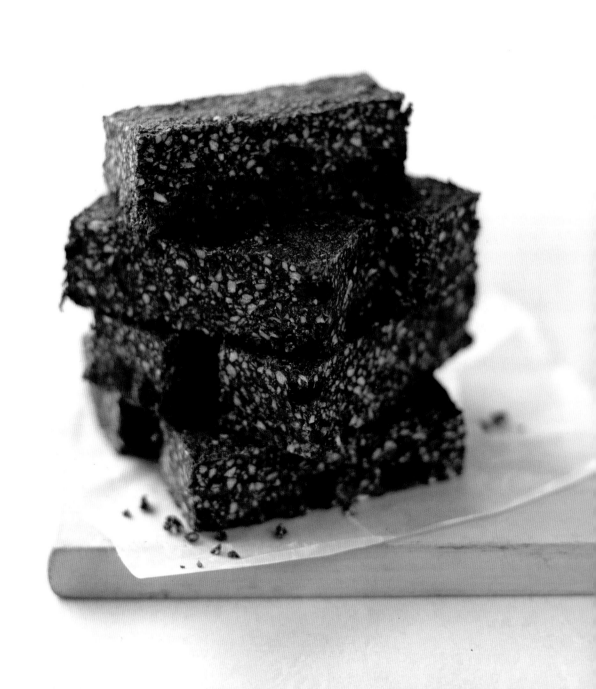

snacks

< black forest cherry bars

A delicious raw protein bar and a great alternative to sugary, shop-bought, processed bars. The combination of protein from the nuts and sweetness from the dried fruit will keep you energized through the day.

SOAKING TIME: *15 minutes* • **PREPARATION TIME:** *30 minutes, plus 1–2 hours chilling time* • **STORAGE:** *will keep in the fridge for up to 1 week. Can freeze for up to 1 month* • **MAKES:** *24 bars*

125g/4½oz/heaped ⅔ cup pitted dates • 150g/5½oz/1½ cups dried cherries • 250g/9oz/1⅔ cups cashew nuts • 250g/9oz/1⅔ cups almonds • 2 tbsp shelled hemp seeds or ground flaxseeds • 85g/3oz/¾ cup raw cacao powder • 150g/5½oz raw cacao butter, melted (see page 17) • 3 tbsp xylitol

1 Soak the dates and half of the dried cherries in warm water for 15 minutes, then drain. Chop the remaining cherries and set aside.
2 Place the nuts in a food processor and process to form a fine meal. Place in a bowl with the hemp seeds and cacao powder.
3 Place the soaked dates and cherries, melted cacao butter and xylitol in a food processor and blend until smooth. Add to the nut mixture with the chopped cherries.
4 Mix thoroughly with your hands to form a stiff dough. Press into a 22cm/8½in square baking tin lined with baking parchment and chill for 1–2 hours until firm, then cut into bars.

HEALTH BENEFITS
*Bursting with **antioxidants**, cherries are a great addition to your raw food diet, helping you feel radiant and energized. Rich in **vitamin C, anthocyanins and quercetin**, they are strongly **anti-inflammatory** and a powerful **immune booster**. Montmorency cherries are particularly rich in **melatonin**, a nutrient important for **promoting sleep**.*

Nutritional analysis per bar: *Calories 223kcal • Protein 5.1g • Carbohydrates 12.3g • Fat 17.5g (of which saturates 5g)*

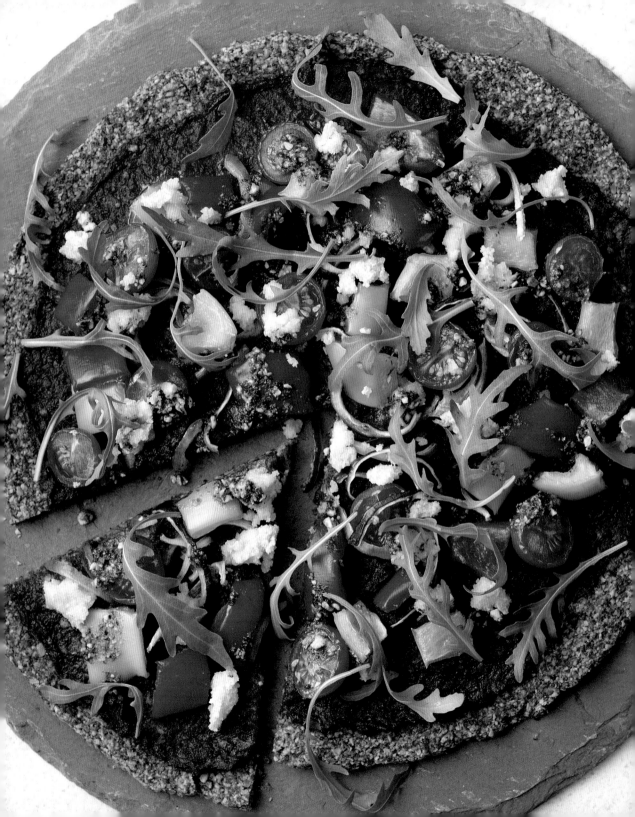

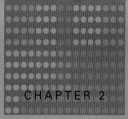

CHAPTER 2

The Raw Food Week Diet

This seven-day Raw Food Week Programme is your key to a slimmer, more radiant you. Whether you are looking to shift stubborn fat, develop a leaner, younger-looking body or gain endless energy, shifting to a raw food diet will get results fast. By the end of the week you should have started to see noticeable weight loss, feel mentally and physically revitalized and be on your way to achieving a glowing, beautiful body.

This is an intensive seven-day programme designed to maximize energy while cleansing your body to enable it to function optimally. I've suggested mouth-watering dishes that are focused on using nutrient-dense, energizing foods. Some take minutes to put together while others may require a little more time but are suitable for preparing ahead. Whether you follow the suggested plan or swap dishes around to suit your tastes, a week in the raw is all you need to experience real results and better health.

< skinny pizza (page 88)

the raw food week programme

It is recommended that you follow this plan after gradually increasing your intake of raw food and experiencing the benefits of the Raw Food Weekend programme.

Start cutting down your consumption of cooked, processed foods and stimulants the week before starting the programme. The night before you start, eat lightly and drink a large glass of warm water and lemon juice. Each day ensure you drink at least 6 glasses (1.5l/52fl oz/6 cups) of plain, filtered water.

Use the seven-day meal plan. By all means swap dishes around, but always include a wide variety of foods throughout the week and plenty of leafy greens each day. Take the daily supplements suggested in the introduction (see page 14).

It is important during the Raw Food Week programme to ensure the majority of your food is raw – ideally 100% but aim for a minimum of 50% of your meals to be raw, with a focus on green leafy vegetables.

Each day make time for breakfast. Start the morning with a glass of warm water and a squeeze of fresh lemon juice, then choose one of the dishes outlined in

the chapter. Try to include green juices and smoothies regularly through the week, ideally daily, either as a breakfast or snack.

Ensure you pack sufficient food for snacks during the day to keep energy levels high and to avoid the temptation to snack on unhealthy options. Nuts, seeds, dehydrated flaxseed crackers, kale chips, smoothies or some fresh fruit are all ideal choices.

Each day either at lunch or dinner make time to have a green leafy salad – these are packed full of essential nutrients and will keep you feeling satisfied for longer. Choose from the suggestions in this chapter and add a delicious raw dressing of your choice.

Whilst I have included a whole range of easy-to-prepare dishes for you, aim to eat simply if you are new to this type of diet. This helps to take the strain out of eating during the week but also ensures correct food combinations, which can avoid digestive upsets and may help the body to process food more efficiently.

During the week, for optimal nutrition without excess calories consume the following foods in abundance:

- Sprouted seeds and beans (see page 20 on sprouting)
- Leafy greens (e.g smoothies, juices, salads, dehydrated kale chips, wraps)
- Slow-releasing low glycemic index fruits (such as berries, apples, pears, plums, apricots, cherries, citrus fruits, peaches and nectarines)
- Sea vegetables (e.g nori wraps, dulse, wakame in salads or sprinkled over raw soups, etc.)

Whilst you need to consume some healthy fats daily, a little goes a long way, so be careful not to overdo your intake of avocados, nuts, seeds and cold-pressed oils. In addition, do not resort to too many sweetened foods or dried fruit, even if they are raw!

Drink plenty of fluids during the day. If you need a warming drink, try herbal or fruit teas or warm water and lemon juice.

It is also recommended that you eat your last meal before 7pm to allow your body sufficient time to digest your food before sleeping. If you feel you need something additional later, then sip a green juice or smoothie. It is important to get adequate rest through the week.

By switching to cleaner, fresher foods, you will be encouraging your body to cleanse itself. This may lead to toxins being released back into the bloodstream in order to be processed by the liver. By ensuring that you get plenty of sleep and rest, you enable the body to regenerate and renew itself, helping you to feel younger from the inside out.

Additionally, include some form of exercise daily. Exercise for at least 30 minutes each day and include a range of different types of exercise, including yoga, pilates for flexibility and relaxation, strength training and cardiovascular exercises such as swimming, running, walking, cycling or cross training. This will stimulate your circulation, aiding detoxification as well as supporting weight loss.

the raw food week plan

day one

On waking A cup of hot water with the juice of ½ lemon

Breakfast Berry Almond Granola (**page 68**) with Almond Milk (**page 24**)

Lunch Mango & Tomato Gazpacho (**page 75**), Flaxseed Crackers (**page 28**) or Courgette Almond Bread (**page 32**), green salad

Snack Flavoured Nut Milk (**page 24**), Cherry & Raspberry Ice (**page 107**)

Dinner Skinny Pizza (**page 88**), Mixed Salad with Caper, Herb & Citrus Dressing (**page 102**)

day two

On waking A cup of hot water with the juice of ½ lemon

Breakfast Fresh Fruit with Citrus & Coconut Cream (**page 67**)

Lunch Creamy Tomato & Apple Dip (**page 76**), Courgette Almond Bread (**page 32**), raw salad of choice, Chocolate-Orange Hazelnut Mousse (**page 108**)

Snack Tomato & Cider Vinegar Kale Chips (**page 104**)

Dinner Vegetable Chilli with Cauliflower 'Rice' (**page 90**)

day three

On waking A cup of hot water with the juice of ½ lemon

Breakfast Pomegranate Superfruits Shake (**page 66**)

Lunch Semi-dried Aubergine Chilli Salad with Sweet Soy Dressing (**page 79**), raw mixed salad, Lucuma & Cinnamon Nuts (**page 30**)

Snack fresh fruit

Dinner Asparagus, Tomato & Basil Quiche (**page 93**), raw mixed salad

day four

On waking A cup of hot water with the juice of ½ lemon

Breakfast Maca & Coconut Power Smoothie (**page 67**)

Lunch Mexican Avocado & Cucumber Soup with Tortilla Chips & Lime Sour Cream (**page 80**)

Snack Spiced Seeds (**page 29**), fresh fruit

Dinner Kelp Noodles with Asian Herbs & Chilli Lime Dressing (**page 95**)

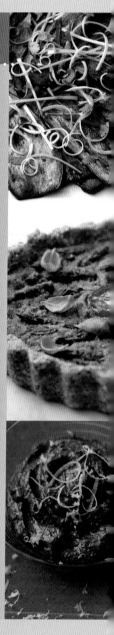

day five

On waking A cup of hot water with the
juice of ½ lemon
Breakfast Vanilla Cream & Peach Parfait
(**page 70**)
Lunch Little Gem Wraps with Herb &
Sun-dried Tomato Pâté (**page 83**),
Flaxseed Crackers (**page 28**), Lemon &
Herb Marinated Olives (**page 27**)
Snack fresh fruit
Dinner Caper Tapenade-Filled
Mushrooms (**page 96**), raw mixed salad

day six

On waking A cup of hot water with the
juice of ½ lemon
Breakfast Chia Coconut Breakfast Bar
(**page 72**)
Lunch Green Papaya Salad with Sweet
Lime Dressing (**page 84**), Toffee Apple
& Carrot Cake (**page 113**)
Snack fresh fruit
Dinner Tamarind Coconut Curry with Fig
& Apple Chutney (**page 98**), Courgette
Almond Bread (**page 32**)

day seven

On waking A cup of hot water with the
juice of ½ lemon
Breakfast Tropical Green Smoothie
(**page 66**), Orange & Apricot Jam with
Raw Bread (**page 71**)
Lunch Summer Greens with Creamy
Pineapple Dressing (**page 87**), Acai
Berry Tart with Lemon Custard
(**page 114**)
Snack Fresh figs with Sweet Nut
Cheese (**page 25**)
Dinner Vegetable Pappardelle with Red
Pepper & Walnut Sauce (**page 101**)

breakfasts

tropical green smoothie

Creamy and rich in energizing essential fats and protein, this smoothie is nourishing and satisfying, yet simple to make.

PREPARATION TIME: *5 minutes* • **STORAGE:** *best drunk immediately* • **SERVES:** *2*

2 large handfuls baby spinach leaves • 375ml/13fl oz/1½ cups coconut water • 2 mangoes, pitted and chopped • 2 tbsp shelled hemp seeds • 1 tbsp xylitol or yacon syrup • 125g/4½fl oz/½ cup crushed ice

1 Place all the ingredients in a blender and blend until smooth.

HEALTH BENEFITS
*Mangoes are rich in **soluble fibre** to keep you feeling fuller for longer, while the **insoluble fibre** aids elimination of waste. A great source of **antioxidants**, including **vitamins C, E and A**, mangoes also help the liver to **remove toxins** from the body.*

Nutritional analysis per serving: *Calories 163kcal • Protein 2.5g • Carbohydrates 34.9g • Fat 2.6g (of which saturates 0.2g)*

pomegranate superfruits shake

This smooth, satisfying juice is rich in protein and essential fats to help keep your metabolism revved up.

PREPARATION TIME: *5 minutes* • **STORAGE:** *best drunk immediately, will keep in the fridge for up to 1 day* • **SERVES:** *2*

250ml/9fl oz/1 cup pure pomegranate juice • 200g/7oz frozen mixed berries • 1 handful sunflower sprouts (optional) • 1 banana, chopped • 2 tsp flaxseed oil

1 Place all the ingredients in a blender with 250ml/9fl oz/1 cup water and blend until smooth.

HEALTH BENEFITS
*A nutrient-dense superfruit, pomegranates are packed with powerful **antioxidants**, including tannins, polyphenols and anthocyanidins, known to **support immune health** and **protect the body** from damaging **free radicals**.*

Nutritional analysis per serving: *Calories 180kcal • Protein 1.8g • Carbohydrates 31.1g • Fat 5.4g (of which saturates 0.5g)*

maca & coconut power smoothie

This smoothie is a delicious way to take in plenty of nutrients, essential fats and phytonutrients.

SOAKING TIME: *2 hours* • **PREPARATION TIME:** *10 minutes + 4 hours or overnight freezing time* • **STORAGE:** *best drunk immediately* • **SERVES:** *2*

---

1 banana, sliced • 60g/2¼oz/scant ½ cup almonds (soaked for 2 hours) • 700ml/24fl oz/2¾ cups coconut water or water • 2 tsp maca powder • 8 pitted dates • ½ tsp green superfood powder • 1 tbsp unsweetened, dried, shredded coconut flakes • 2 tsp raw cacao powder • 1 tsp lecithin powder

1 Put the banana in a lidded container and freeze for 4 hours or overnight.
2 Place all the ingredients in a blender and blend until smooth and creamy.

HEALTH BENEFITS
Rich in **amino acids,** *maca root is a popular raw superfood, sometimes referred to as "Peruvian ginseng". Known as an* **adaptogen,** *it is useful in helping the body to* **cope with stress, elevate mood** *and* **improve endurance.**

Nutritional analysis per serving: *Calories 384kcal • Protein 9.3g • Carbohydrates 37.4g • Fat 20.3g (of which saturates 2g)*

fresh fruit with citrus & coconut cream

An easy-to-assemble breakfast, or a delicious snack during the day.

PREPARATION TIME: *depending on the fruits used, about 15 minutes* • **STORAGE:** *the cream can be prepared in advance and kept in the fridge for up to 2 days* • **SERVES:** *4*

---

a selection of prepared fresh fruits, such as pineapple, mango and lychees

CITRUS & COCONUT CREAM: 125g/4½oz/ heaped ¾ cup macadamia nuts • 2 tbsp unsweetened, dried, shredded coconut flakes • 1 tbsp coconut butter, melted (see page 17) • 4 dates • zest and juice of 3 oranges • zest of 1 lemon

1 Place the cream ingredients in a blender and blend until smooth. Add a little water to thin, if necessary. Serve with the fresh fruit.

HEALTH BENEFITS
Coconut increases the **burning of calories.**

Nutritional analysis per serving: *Calories 319kcal • Protein 3.2g • Carbohydrates 9.7g • Fat 29.7g (of which saturates 6.8g)*

berry almond granola >

This amazing raw food granola is delicious and nutritious for breakfast or as a snack. Ensure it is thoroughly dried before storing it in an airtight container.

SOAKING TIME: *2 hours* • **PREPARATION TIME:** *15 minutes* • **DEHYDRATING TIME:** *17 hours* • **STORAGE:** *will keep in an airtight container for up to 1 week* • **SERVES:** *8*

270g/9½oz/1½ cups pitted dates • 40g/1½oz melted coconut butter (see page 17) • 140g/5oz/scant 1 cup almonds (soaked for 2 hours) • 60g/2¼oz/heaped ⅓ cup Brazil nuts (soaked for 2 hours) • 125g/4½oz/heaped ⅔ cup pumpkin seeds (soaked for 2 hours) • 125g/4½oz/1 cup sunflower seeds (soaked for 2 hours) • 1 apple, peeled and diced • ½ tsp cinnamon • ½ tsp sea salt • 85g/3oz/heaped ½ cup dried cherries, blueberries and cranberries

1 Place the dates and the coconut butter in a food processor with 125ml/4fl oz/½ cup water and blend to form a stiff paste.
2 Drain all the nuts and seeds. Place in a food processor and pulse lightly to form small pieces. Do not over-process.
3 Place the nuts and seeds in a large bowl and add the paste, apple, cinnamon and salt. Mix well by hand to ensure all the mixture is thoroughly coated with the paste.
4 Scatter the mixture over a non-stick sheet placed on a baking or dehydrator tray. Put in a dehydrator set at 45°C/115°F, or place in an oven at 45°C/115°F (or on its lowest setting with the door ajar), for 17 hours until crisp. Stir in the berries.

HEALTH BENEFITS
*Brazil nuts are one of the richest sources of the antioxidant **selenium**, a trace mineral known to protect the body from **oxidative stress and cancerous cells**. It is also needed for the production of **glutathione**, which plays an important role in **minimizing free radical damage** and **immune health**. It also helps the proper functioning of the **thyroid gland**, important for **controlling metabolism**. Brazil nuts are also high in **protein** and **fibre** so can help to **control hunger**, boosting **weight loss**.*

Nutritional analysis per serving: *Calories 490kcal • Protein 12.7g • Carbohydrates 35.3g • Fat 32.8g (of which saturates 8.1g)*

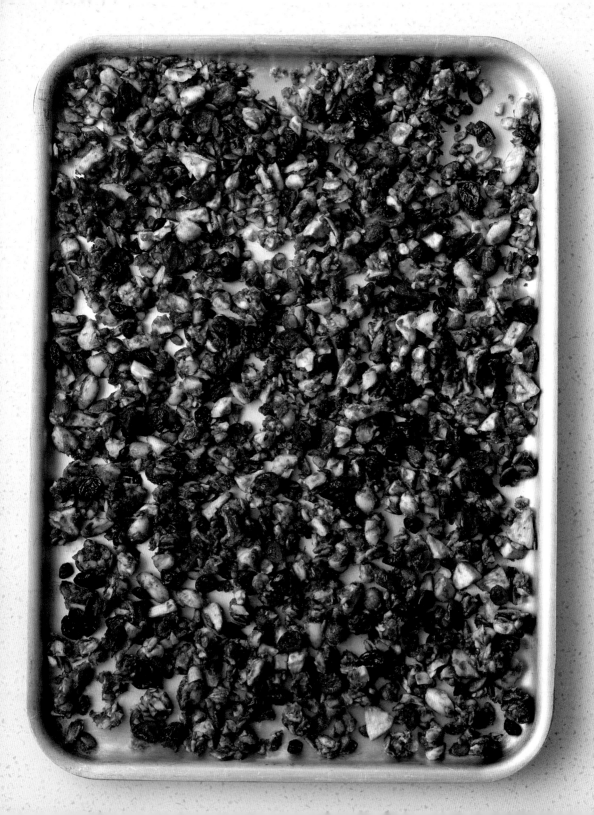

vanilla cream & peach parfait

A healthy raw version of "peaches and cream", this is a simple, satisfying breakfast treat and equally delicious as a pudding or sweet snack. Layers of vanilla cream coat slices of peaches and fresh raspberries, but you could serve the cream with other fruits, depending on the season.

PREPARATION TIME: *15 minutes* • **STORAGE:** *the cream will keep in the fridge for up to 3–4 days* • **SERVES:** *6*

3 peaches, halved, pitted and sliced • 250g/9oz/2 cups raspberries

VANILLA CREAM: 2 tbsp vanilla extract • 250ml/9fl oz/1 cup coconut water • 300g/10½oz/scant 2 cups pine nuts or cashew nuts • 4 tbsp xylitol or other sweetener

1 To make the vanilla cream, place all the ingredients in a blender and blend until smooth.
2 Place slices of peach in the bottom of each of 6 glasses and top with a handful of raspberries. Spoon a layer of the vanilla cream on top and repeat the layering.
3 Top each glass with a couple of raspberries to serve.

HEALTH BENEFITS
*If you need a quick pick-me-up, peaches make a healthy, low-calorie boost. A great source of the antioxidants **beta-carotene** and **vitamin C**, they will also nourish your **immune system** and keep you feeling **energized** throughout the morning.*

Nutritional analysis per serving: *Calories 343kcal • Protein 6.8g • Carbohydrates 18.8g • Fat 28.7g (of which saturates 2g)*

orange & apricot jam
with raw bread

An easy, raw version of toast and jam, but much more nutritious. You can soak the apricots overnight in the orange juice to save time, or make the jam in advance and store it in the fridge.

SOAKING TIME: *1 hour* • **PREPARATION TIME:** *10 minutes* • **STORAGE:** *the jam will keep in the fridge for up to 1 week. It can be frozen for up to 1 month* • **MAKES:** *12 servings of jam*

175g/6oz/scant 1 cup dried apricots • juice and zest of 2 oranges • 1 slice Courgette Almond Bread (see page 32) or 2 Date or Raisin Crackers (see page 28), to serve

1 Place the apricots and orange juice and zest in a bowl and leave to soak for 1 hour. Purée with a hand-held blender or using a food processor to form a stiff paste.
2 Spread a little of the jam on the raw bread or crackers to serve.

HEALTH BENEFITS
*Dried apricots, like other dried fruits, are a concentrated source of **nutrients** and **natural sugars**, making them the perfect pick-me-up sweet treat. Apricots are particularly rich in **beta-carotene**, **iron, potassium, calcium and magnesium**. Iron is needed for **haemoglobin production**, making it useful for tackling fatigue or flagging energy levels.*

Nutritional analysis per tablespoon of jam • *Calories 19kcal* • *Protein 0.5g* • *Carbohydrates 4.1g* • *Fat 0.1g (of which saturates 0g)*

chia coconut breakfast bars >

These are perfect for when you need something quick. A delicious tropical combination of dried mango and coconut, these bars are simple and easy to prepare. Chia seeds are a great way to boost your intake of omega-3 fats.

SOAKING TIME: *10 minutes* • **PREPARATION TIME:** *30 minutes, plus 2 hours chilling time*
• **STORAGE:** *will keep in the fridge for up to 1 week. Can be frozen for up to 1 month* • **MAKES:** *18 bars*

200g/7oz/heaped 1¼ cups almonds • 2 heaped tbsp chia seeds • 125g/4½oz/2 cups dried mango, chopped (soaked for 10 minutes, then drained) • juice of 1 orange • 2 tbsp xylitol • 4 tbsp melted coconut butter (see page 17) • pinch sea salt • 3 tbsp lucuma powder • 40g/1½oz/heaped ⅓ cup ground flaxseeds • 120g/4¼oz/1⅓ cups desiccated coconut

1 Place the almonds in a blender and blend to a fine flour. Repeat with the chia seeds.
2 Place half the mango in a blender with the chia powder, orange juice, xylitol, melted coconut butter and salt. Blend to form a thick purée. Finely chop the remaining mango.
3 Place the ground almonds, lucuma powder, ground flaxseeds, mango pieces and three-quarters of the coconut in a large bowl. Pour in the purée and stir until blended.
4 Sprinkle a little of the reserved coconut over the base of a baking parchment-lined traybake tin, about 30 x 20cm/12 x 8in. Press the mixture into the tin and flatten the surface. Sprinkle the remaining coconut on top, pressing down firmly. Chill for 2 hours until firm, then cut into bars.

HEALTH BENEFITS
*Chia seeds are an amazingly nutritious dieter's superfood, rich in **essential omega-3 fatty acids** and **antioxidants**, which protect these healthy fats from being oxidized. Chia seeds also provide plenty of **fibre** as well as **calcium, phosphorus, magnesium, manganese, copper, iron, molybdenum, niacin and zinc**. When chia seeds are added to water, they form a gel that helps to slow down the digestion of sugars, helping to **stabilize blood sugar** and keeping you **feeling fuller** for longer.*

Nutritional analysis per bar: *Calories 209kcal • Protein 3.6g • Carbohydrates 12.8g • Fat 16.1g (of which saturates 7.8g)*

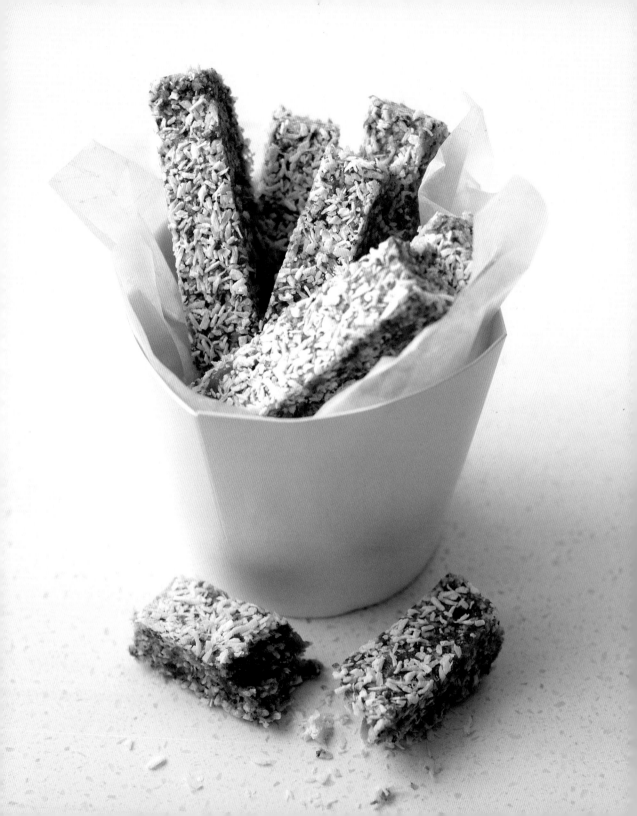

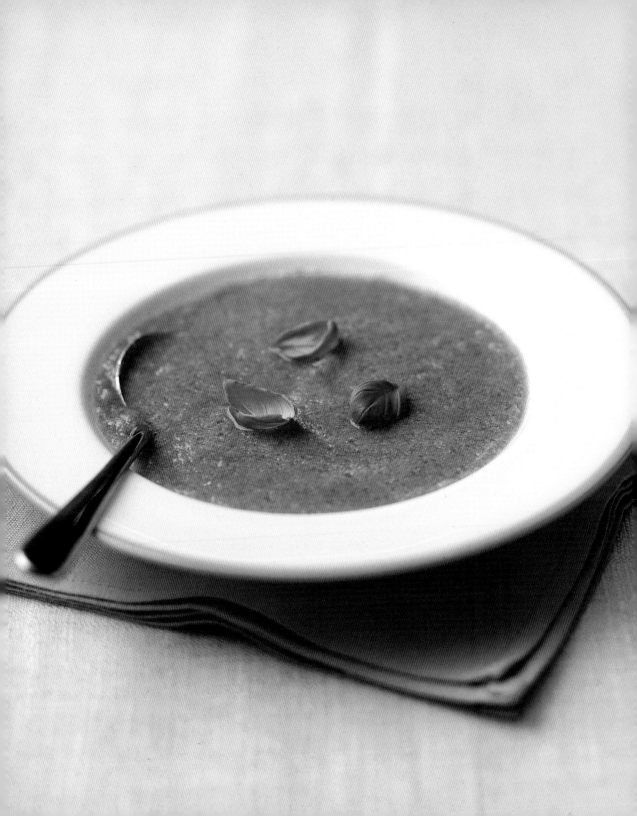

lunches

< mango & tomato gazpacho

This refreshing soup, served with a slice of raw bread or flaxseed crackers, is perfect for a light lunch. The mango adds a wonderful sweet, tropical flavour to the soup and is a great way to boost your intake of antioxidants, too. If possible, prepare the soup the day before to allow the flavours to develop.

PREPARATION TIME: *20 minutes, plus 2 hours chilling time* • **STORAGE**: *will keep in the fridge for up to 3 days* • **SERVES**: *4*

450g/1lb ripe plum tomatoes, chopped • **¼ white onion, chopped** • **1 red pepper, halved lengthways, deseeded and chopped** • **1 garlic clove, minced** • **1 tbsp sherry vinegar** • **1 ripe mango, pitted and cubed** • **½ tsp sea salt** • **freshly ground black pepper** • **a few basil leaves, to scatter** • **1 slice Courgette Almond Bread (see page 32) or 2 Date or Raisin Crackers (see page 28), to serve**

1 Place all the ingredients in a blender and blend until smooth.
2 Press the soup through a sieve into a large bowl and season with salt and pepper to taste.
3 Chill for 2 hours, then spoon into bowls, scatter with the basil leaves and serve with the raw bread or crackers.

HEALTH BENEFITS
*Onions are a superb **cleansing** and **weight-loss** food – rich in **sulphur** to support **liver function** and help **clear out toxins** from the body. They also contain **allicin** and other powerful natural **antibiotics** that help fight off **infections** and support **immune function**.*

Nutritional analysis per serving: Calories 49kcal • Protein 1.3g • Carbohydrates 9.7g • Fat 0.5g
(of which saturates 0.2g)

creamy tomato & apple dip >

This delicious raw dip is naturally sweet and packed full of flavour, using a combination of apple and fresh and sun-dried tomatoes. It is perfect as a snack with vegetable sticks or raw crackers, or as part of a light lunch.

SOAKING TIME: *2 hours* • **PREPARATION TIME:** *10 minutes* • **STORAGE:** *will keep in the fridge for up to 3–4 days*

115g/4oz/¾ cup pine nuts (soaked for 2 hours, then drained) • 1 apple, peeled, cored and quartered • 1 tomato, chopped • 4 sun-dried tomatoes • 1 tbsp extra virgin olive oil • 2 tsp tamari soy sauce • 1 tbsp apple cider vinegar • sea salt • freshly ground black pepper • vegetable sticks or Flaxseed Crackers (see page 28), to serve (optional)

1 Place all the ingredients in a food processor and process until creamy, adding a little water as needed to thin. Season with salt and pepper to taste.
2 Transfer to a bowl and serve with vegetable sticks or crackers.

HEALTH BENEFITS
*Pine nuts are a dieter's dream – a great source of **pinolenic acid**, which is thought to stimulate hormones that help to **diminish your appetite**. They are also rich in **oleic acid**, a monounsaturated fat shown to **lower harmful fats** in the body and protect the **heart**. They are packed with **iron** and **magnesium** – useful minerals for **maintaining energy and alleviating fatigue**.*

Nutritional analysis per tablespoon: *Calories 54kcal • Protein 0.9g • Carbohydrates 0.8g • Fat 5.2g (of which saturates 0.4g)*

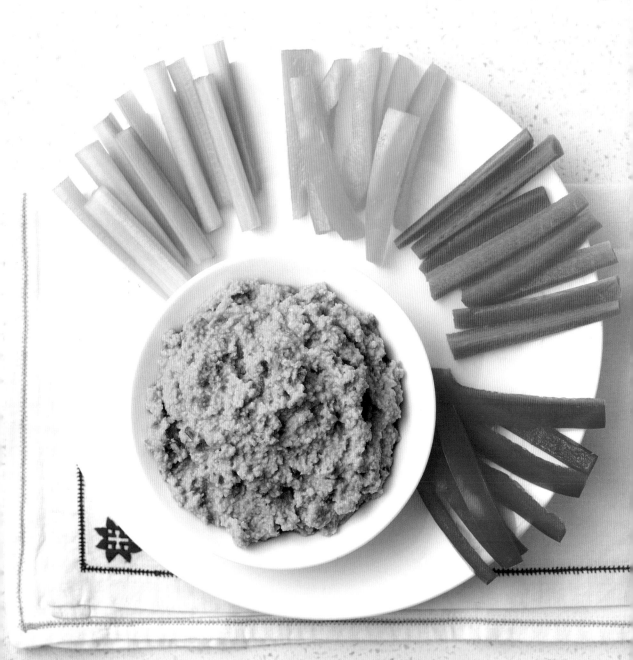

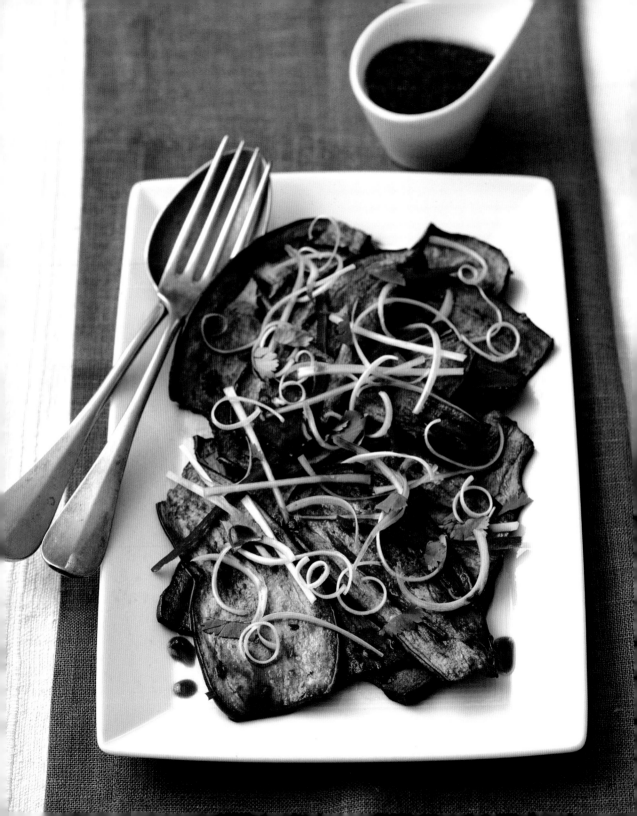

< semi-dried aubergine chilli salad with sweet soy dressing

A wonderful Japanese-inspired dish with marinated, dehydrated aubergines taking centre stage. The sweet soy dressing is equally delicious served as a dipping sauce or drizzled over pak choi or other greens.

PREPARATION TIME: *15 minutes, plus 1 hour marinating time* • **DEHYDRATING TIME:** *3–4 hours* • **STORAGE:** *the marinade/dressing will keep in the fridge for up to 2–3 days* • **SERVES:** *4*

---

2 small aubergines • 1 red chilli, deseeded and julienned • 4 spring onions, cut into thin strips • 1 handful coriander leaves, chopped

MARINADE: 5 tbsp tamari soy sauce • 3 tbsp xylitol, yacon syrup or coconut nectar • 1 garlic clove, minced • juice of 1 lime • 1 red chilli, deseeded and finely chopped • 1 tbsp rice vinegar • 2 tbsp extra virgin olive oil

1 Thinly slice the aubergines lengthways with a knife or mandolin slicer.
2 To make the marinade, mix together all the ingredients in a bowl. Pour over the aubergines and leave to marinate for 1 hour.
3 Drain the aubergine slices, reserving the marinade, and place on a non-stick sheet placed on a baking or dehydrator tray. Put in a dehydrator set at 45°C/115°F for 3–4 hours until semi-dry but still soft. Alternatively, place in an oven at 45°C/115°F (or on its lowest setting with the door ajar) for 3 hours.
4 Place the aubergine slices on a large plate and scatter with the chilli, spring onions and coriander leaves. Use the reserved marinade as a dressing to serve.

HEALTH BENEFITS
Chillies help to *suppress appetite, regulate blood sugar levels* and *boost metabolism. They are a great source of **beta-carotene** and **vitamins C** and **E**, and contain **folic acid and potassium**.*

Nutritional analysis per serving: *Calories 121kcal • Protein 1.7g • Carbohydrates 15.1g • Fat 7.9g (of which saturates 1.2g)*

mexican avocado & cucumber soup with lime sour cream >

A light, mildly spiced soup, topped with a refreshing protein-rich cream to keep you satisfied throughout the afternoon. Serve with tortilla or corn chips.

PREPARATION TIME: *20 minutes* • **DEHYDRATING TIME:** *20 minutes (optional)* • **STORAGE:** *best eaten immediately. The cream will keep in the fridge for up to 2–3 days* • **SERVES:** *4*

1 large ripe avocado, halved, pitted and chopped • ½ cucumber, peeled • 1 spring onion, chopped • juice of 1 lime • 2 tbsp coriander leaves • 3 ripe plum tomatoes, chopped • pinch of chilli powder • ½ tsp ground cumin • ½ tsp ground coriander • ½ tsp sea salt • 250ml/9fl oz/1 cup coconut water or water • 8–12 Tortilla or Corn Chips, to serve (see page 31)

LIME SOUR CREAM: 115g/4oz/¾ cup pine nuts • 185ml/6fl oz/¾ cup coconut water or water • juice of 1 lime • 1 tomato • 1 tbsp xylitol (optional) • 1 garlic clove • ½ tsp sea salt

1 To make the lime sour cream, place all the ingredients in a blender and blend until smooth. Place in a bowl and chill until needed.
2 Place the soup ingredients in a food processor and process until smooth. Warm in a bowl in a dehydrator or low oven for 20 minutes, if you like.
3 Spoon the soup into bowls and drizzle with a spoonful of the lime sour cream. Serve with tortilla or corn chips.

HEALTH BENEFITS

*Avocados are a great source of healthy **monounsaturated fat**, plus they contain **protein** to help balance **blood sugar levels**, making them useful for preventing energy dips and cravings later in the day. They are also rich in **anti-ageing antioxidants** (vitamins A, C and E) and contain **potassium** for reducing fluid retention, as well as **energizing, anti-stress B vitamins**.*

Nutritional analysis per serving (soup and 1 tbsp cream): *Calories 102kcal • Protein 1.9g • Carbohydrates 5.7g • Fat 7.9g (of which saturates 1.3g)*

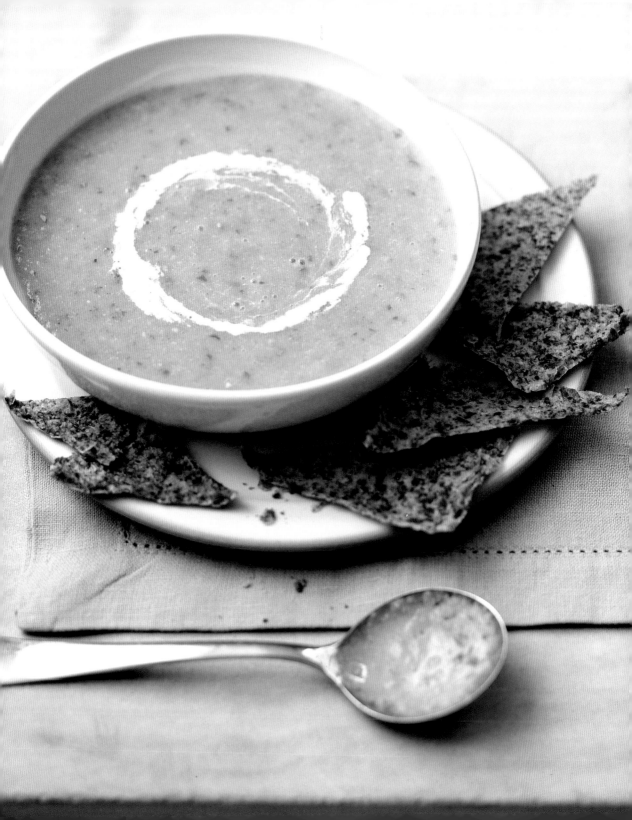

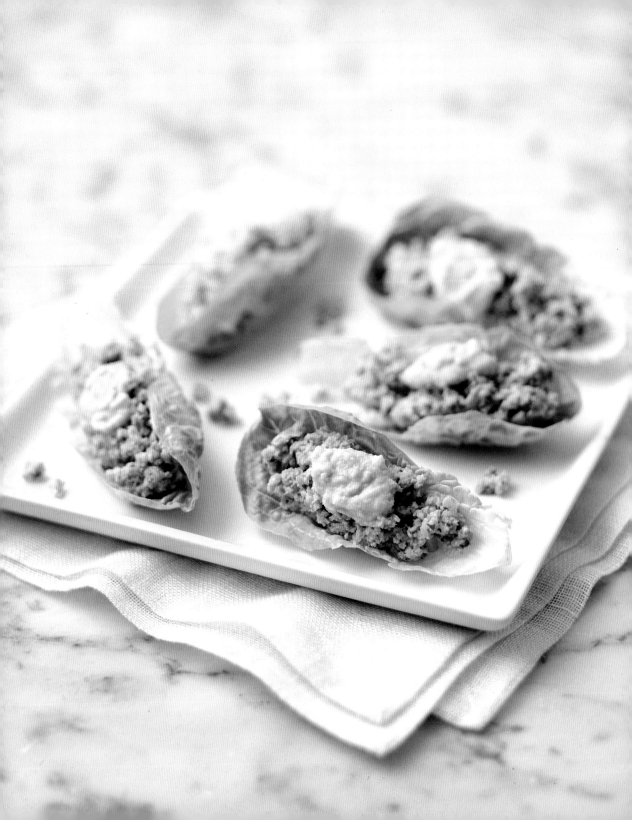

< little gem wraps with herb & sun-dried tomato pâté

A summery herb pâté packed with protein to keep hunger pangs at bay. This is delicious used as a topping for crackers, raw breads and vegetables, as well as being the perfect filling for wraps and sushi rolls.

SOAKING TIME: *2–3 hours or overnight* • **PREPARATION TIME:** *15 minutes* • **STORAGE:** *the pâté will keep in the fridge for up to 2–3 days* • **SERVES:** *4*

125g/4½oz/1 cup sunflower seeds (soaked for 2–3 hours or overnight, then drained) • 60g/2¼oz/heaped ⅓ cup almonds (soaked for 2–3 hours or overnight, then drained) • 1 tbsp chopped dill, • 2 tbsp chopped parsley • 1 tbsp chopped basil leaves • juice and zest of ½ lemon • 1 tsp sea salt • 2 tbsp extra virgin olive oil or flaxseed oil • freshly ground black pepper • 2 celery sticks, finely chopped • 1 garlic clove, minced • 6 sun-dried tomatoes, chopped • 4 Little Gem lettuces, leaves separated • 4 tbsp Vegan Nut Mayonnaise (see page 26), to serve (optional)

1 Place the sunflower seeds and almonds in a food processor and process to form small pieces. Add the rest of the ingredients, except the Little Gems, and process to form a chunky pâté.
2 Place a spoonful on to each Little Gem leaf and top with a small amount of nut mayonnaise, if you like.

HEALTH BENEFITS
*Parsley is a great **cleansing** food and a wonderful **diuretic** to help tackle fluid retention, making it a useful addition to your weight-loss programme. It is also rich in nutrients, including **vitamin K**, **iron** and **folate**, and in **antioxidants**, including **vitamin C and beta-carotene**.*

Nutritional analysis per serving: *Calories 419kcal • Protein 11.3g • Carbohydrates 8g • Fat 37.2g (of which saturates 4.9g)*

green papaya salad with sweet lime dressing >

Green, or unripe, papaya are long, green fruits now readily available in supermarkets and Asian shops. This Thai-style salad is light and fragrant, and the strips of papaya and carrot soak up the delicious lime dressing beautifully.

PREPARATION TIME: *15 minutes + marinating* • **STORAGE:** *the salad can be kept in the fridge for up to 2 days and the dressing for up to 4 days* • **SERVES:** *2*

---

1 large green papaya, seeds and soft centre discarded, julienned • 2 spring onions, chopped • 2 carrots, julienned • ½ cucumber, deseeded and julienned • handful basil or Thai basil leaves • handful mint leaves • handful coriander leaves • 40g/1¼oz/¼ cup chopped almonds

DRESSING: juice of 2 limes • 1 tbsp xylitol • 1 garlic clove, minced • 1 tbsp chopped coriander • 2 tsp tamari soy sauce • ½ red chilli, deseeded and chopped

1 To make the salad, place the papaya in a large bowl with the spring onions, carrots and cucumber.
2 To make the dressing, put all the ingredients in a bowl and mix together.
3 Drizzle the dressing over the salad and toss well. Leave to marinate for 15 minutes then toss again. Add the herbs and almonds before serving.

HEALTH BENEFITS
*Fresh herbs add a wonderful flavour to salads and dishes and are also packed with **nutrients** and possess many health-promoting properties. Rich in **antioxidants**, particularly **flavonoids**, they help to protect the body against pollutants and toxins. Their fragrant volatile oils possess **anti-microbial activity**, making them useful for protecting against unwanted bacteria, fungi and parasites.*

Nutritional analysis per serving: *Calories 193kcal • Protein 6.4g • Carbohydrates 18.4g • Fat 15.5g (of which saturates 0.9g)*

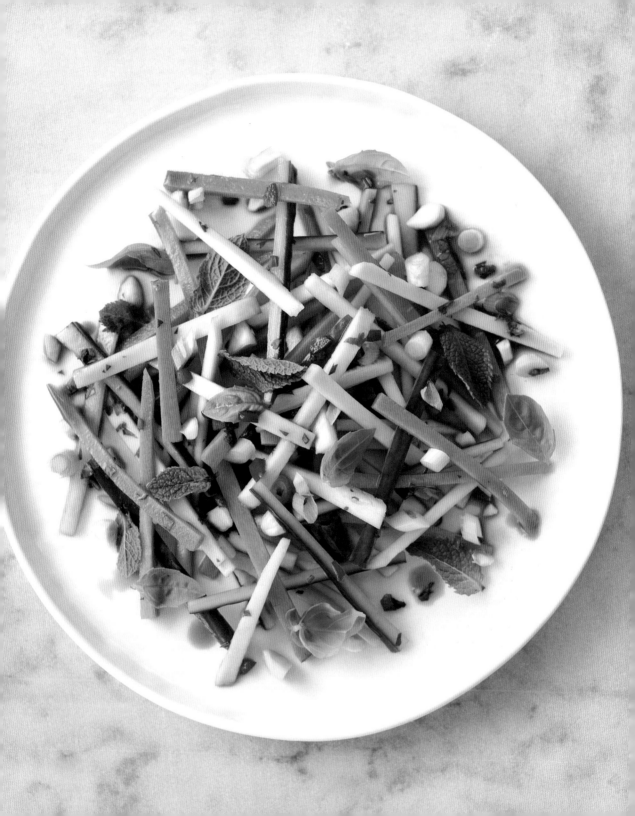

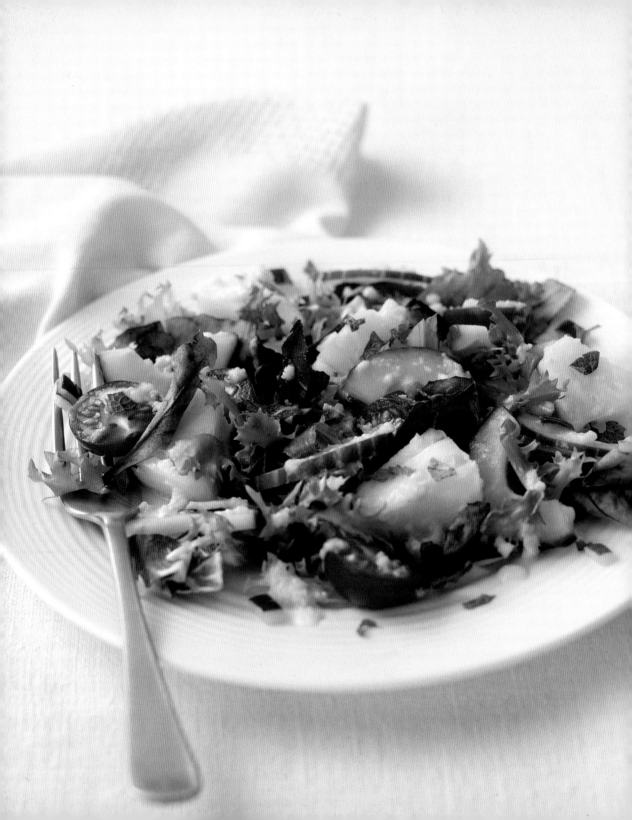

< summer greens with creamy pineapple dressing

The wonderful sweet and tangy flavours of the dressing are guaranteed to liven up any salad. The addition of pine nuts creates a delicious creamy texture, while keeping the dish light and fresh.

SOAKING TIME: *15 minutes* • **PREPARATION TIME:** *15 minutes* • **STORAGE:** *the dressing will keep in the fridge for up to 2–3 days* • **SERVES:** *4*

300g/10½oz mixed salad leaves • ¼ pineapple, cored and cut into chunks • 1 handful mixed sprouted seeds (optional) • 150g/5½oz cherry tomatoes, halved • 1 tbsp chopped mint leaves • 1 small red onion, diced • ½ cucumber, deseeded and sliced

PINEAPPLE DRESSING: 30g/1oz/½ cup dried pineapple (soaked for 15 minutes, then drained) • 30g/1oz/scant ¼ cup pine nuts • 2 tbsp lemon juice • 1 tsp Dijon mustard • 1 garlic clove, minced • 185ml/6fl oz/¾ cup coconut water or water • ½ tsp sea salt • freshly ground black pepper

1 To make the dressing, place the dried pineapple in a blender with the remaining dressing ingredients and blend until smooth.
2 Place all the salad ingredients in a large bowl and mix together. Just before serving, toss with the dressing.

HEALTH BENEFITS
*The **menthol** in peppermint is well known to **soothe the digestive tract** and help **relieve flatulence and indigestion**. It also promotes the secretion of digestive juices and has calming and **anti-inflammatory** properties to **soothe an irritable bowel**.*

Nutritional analysis per serving: *Calories 132kcal • Protein 3.4g • Carbohydrates 15.5g • Fat 6.1g (of which saturates 0.5g)*

dinners

skinny pizza >

A delicious, healthy, raw version of the popular fast food, which can be
prepared in advance and warmed through before serving. This version
includes simple Mediterranean flavours, but do feel free to vary the toppings.

PREPARATION TIME: *45 minutes* • **DEHYDRATING TIME:** *2–3 hours* • **STORAGE:** *the remaining pesto
will keep in the fridge for up to 3–4 days* • **SERVES:** *6*

½ **recipe quantity Sun-Dried Tomato Sauce (see page 27) • 1 Pizza Base (see page 33)**
• ½ **red onion, sliced** • ½ **red pepper, deseeded and cut into chunks** • ½ **yellow pepper,
deseeded and cut into chunks** • **8 cherry tomatoes, halved** • **4 tbsp Basic Nut Cheese
(see page 25)** • **1 large handful rocket or watercress leaves, to serve**

PISTACHIO PESTO: 40g/1½oz/**heaped 1 cup basil leaves** • 70g/2½oz/**scant ½ cup
pistachio nuts** • **4–6 tbsp extra virgin olive oil or flaxseed oil** • ¼ **tsp sea salt**
• **1 garlic clove, minced** • **2 tsp lemon juice** • **1 tbsp dried nutritional yeast flakes**

1 Place all the pesto ingredients in a blender and blend to form a smooth paste.
2 Spread a little of the tomato sauce over the pizza base. Top with the onion, red and
   yellow pepper and tomatoes. Dot with the nut cheese and drizzle over half of the pesto.
3 Place on a baking or dehydrator tray. Warm through in a dehydrator or cool oven for
   2–3 hours before serving. Scatter with rocket leaves to serve.

HEALTH BENEFITS
*Packed with nutrients, **watercress** and **rocket** are fantastic supergreens to add to your raw
food diet. Low in calories and a useful diuretic, they can help **reduce fluid retention** and tackle
bloating. They are also packed with **minerals** and **liver-supporting nutrients** to aid the **elimination
of toxins** and speed up **fat loss**.*

Nutritional analysis per serving: *Calories 409kcal • Protein 10.1g • Carbohydrates 15.3g • Fat 34.7g
(of which saturates 3.9g)*

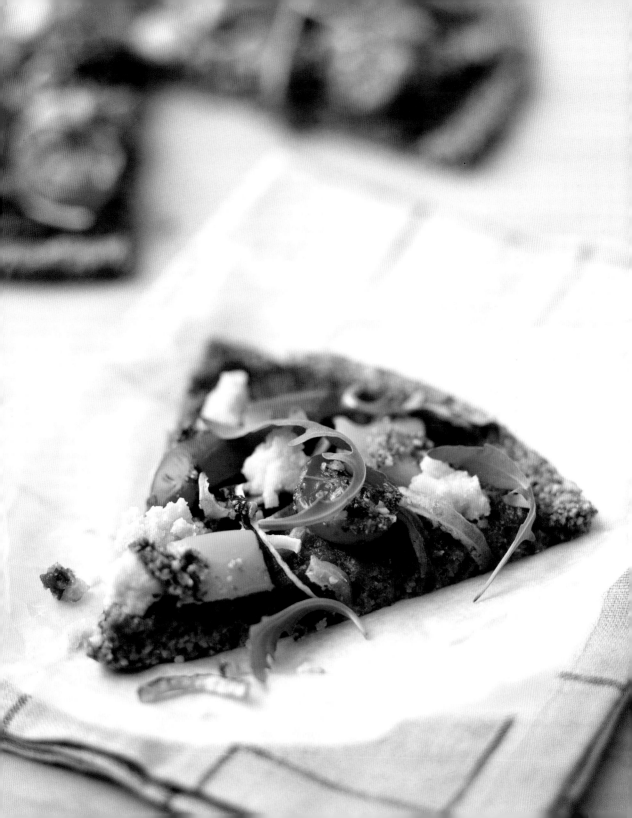

vegetable chilli with cauliflower "rice" >

Adding a selection of mushrooms to this chilli provides not only a wonderful texture but protein too. Shiitake mushrooms are also a good source of iron. The chocolate-chilli sauce would also work well for dipping corn chips.

PREPARATION TIME: *30 minutes* • **DEHYDRATING TIME:** *1 hour* • **STORAGE:** *will keep in the fridge for up to 2 days* • **SERVES:** *4*

½ cauliflower, cut into florets • 30g/1oz/¼ cup pine nuts • ½ tsp sea salt • freshly ground black pepper • juice of ½ lemon • 2 tsp tahini • 1 red pepper, deseeded and chopped • 1 yellow pepper, deseeded and chopped • 2 tomatoes, chopped • 8 chestnut mushrooms, chopped • 6 shiitake mushrooms, chopped • 1 courgette, diced • 2 spring onions, chopped • 1 tbsp chopped coriander

SAUCE: 1 recipe quantity Sun-dried Tomato Sauce (see page 27) • 1 tbsp raw cacao powder • 1 garlic clove, minced • pinch smoked paprika • ½ tsp deseeded and chopped red chilli • pinch sea salt

1 Place the cauliflower, pine nuts, salt, pepper, lemon juice and tahini in a food processor and process to form rice-like grains. Place in a bowl.
2 Blend the sauce ingredients in a blender until smooth. Add a little water if needed.
3 Place the remaining ingredients in a separate bowl and pour the sauce over the top. Warm in a dehydrator or cool oven with the bowl of rice for 1 hour before serving.

HEALTH BENEFITS
*Cauliflowers, like other vegetables in the brassica family, are rich in **cancer-fighting sulphurous compounds**, which also **support liver function** and **detoxification**. They are also a great source of **B vitamins**, including **folate**, which is an important **heart-protective** nutrient.*

Nutritional analysis per serving: *Calories 236kcal • Protein 7.2g • Carbohydrates 15.8g • Fat 15.8g (of which saturates 2g)*

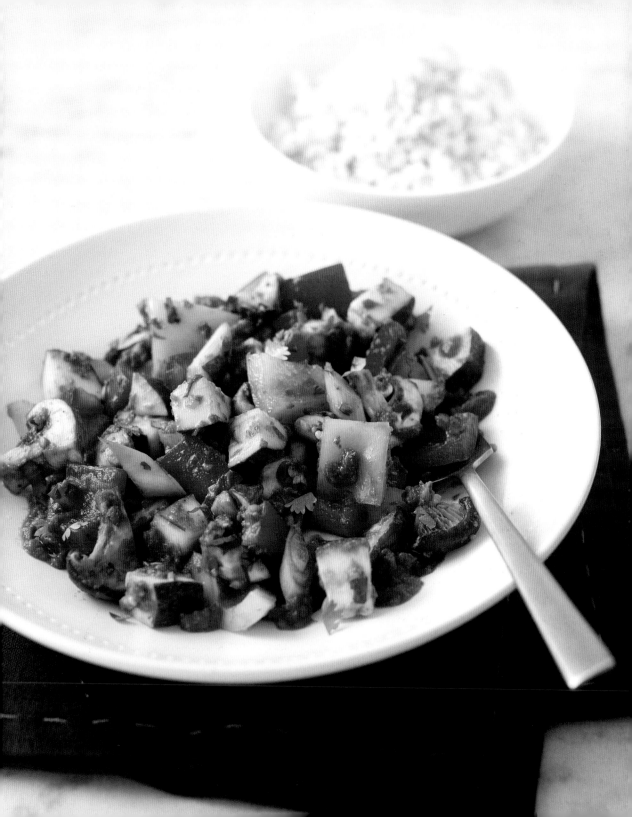

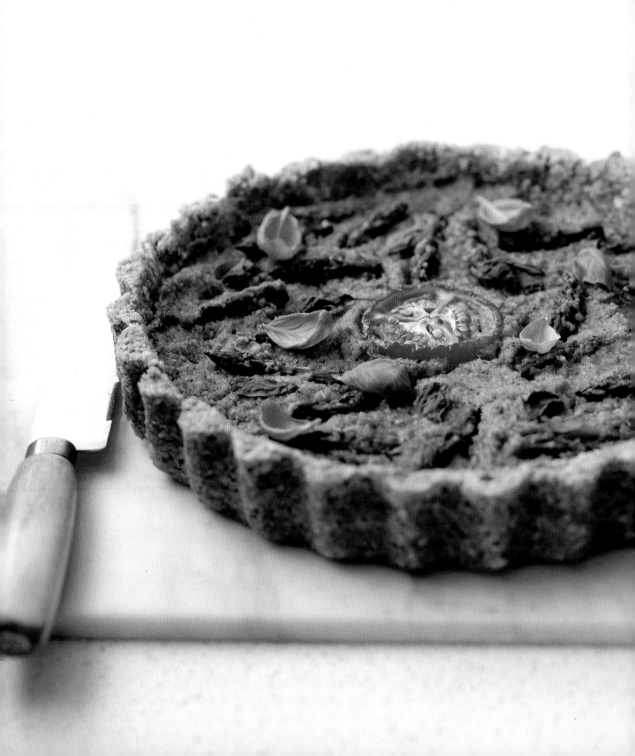

< asparagus, tomato & basil quiche

This creamy, satisfying raw tart is full of light, spring flavours.

SOAKING TIME: *2 hours* ● **PREPARATION TIME:** *30 minutes* ● **DEHYDRATING TIME:** *8 hours*
● **STORAGE:** *will keep in the fridge for up to 2–3 days* ● **SERVES:** *6–8*

125g/4½oz/heaped ¾ cup cashew nuts (soaked for 2 hours, then drained) ● 115g/4oz/
heaped ⅔ cup whole flaxseeds ● 1 courgette, chopped ● ½ tsp sea salt ● 1 tbsp dried
nutritional yeast flakes ● 4 tbsp melted coconut butter (see page 17)

FILLING: 1 courgette, chopped ● 115g/4oz/¾ cup pine nuts ● pinch sea salt ● 1 garlic
clove, minced ● 2 tbsp dried nutritional yeast flakes ● 100g/3½oz/⅔ cup sun-dried
tomatoes, soaked for 30 minutes, then drained and chopped ● 100g/3½oz/1 cup
chopped asparagus tips ● slice of tomato ● 1 handful basil leaves, to scatter

1 Place the cashew nuts and flaxseeds in a blender and blend until fine. Tip into a bowl.
2 Put the courgette, salt, yeast flakes and coconut butter in the blender and blend until
   smooth. Add to the nuts and mix to form the pastry, adding a little water if needed.
   Press into a greased 23cm/9in tart or pie dish.
3 Put in a dehydrator set at 45°C/115°F, or place in an oven at 45°C/115°F (or on its
   lowest setting with the door ajar) for 4 hours or until dry at the edges.
4 To make the filling, blend the courgette, pine nuts, salt, garlic, yeast flakes, half the
   sun-dried tomatoes and 125ml/4fl oz/½ cup water in a food processor until creamy.
5 Stir in the asparagus tips and remaining sun-dried tomatoes. Spread the mixture
   evenly over the crust. Put the slice of tomato in the centre. Warm in the dehydrator
   or cool oven for 4 hours. Scatter with basil leaves before serving.

HEALTH BENEFITS
*Asparagus is an effective **diuretic**. Its **cleansing** and **anti-inflammatory** properties make it useful
for reducing **oedema** and **fluid retention** and easing the symptoms of **arthritis**.*

Nutritional analysis per serving (for 6): *Calories 425kcal ● Protein 11.6g ● Carbohydrates 11.3g
● Fat 37.9g (of which saturates 10.1g)*

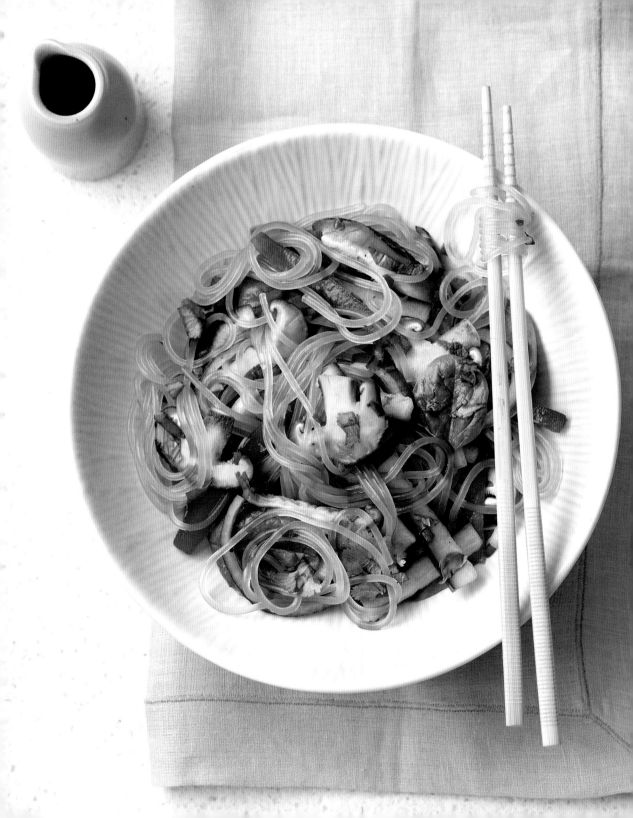

< kelp noodles with asian herbs & chilli lime dressing

Kelp noodles are low in calories, can be used instead of wheat pasta and are totally unprocessed. Marinating the vegetables in the Asian-spiced dressing enhances the flavour and creates a soft, more "cooked" texture.

SOAKING TIME: *20 minutes* • **PREPARATION TIME:** *20 minutes* • **STORAGE:** *will keep in the fridge for up to 1 day* • **SERVES:** *4*

½ **red onion, thinly sliced** • **225g/8oz/1½ cups shiitake mushrooms, sliced** • **1 red pepper, halved lengthways, deseeded and julienned** • ½ **cucumber, deseeded and julienned** • **1 tbsp chopped Thai basil leaves** • **1 tbsp chopped mint leaves** • **1 tbsp chopped coriander leaves** • **1 large handful baby spinach leaves** • **350g/12oz kelp noodles (soaked for 20 minutes, then drained)**

CHILLI LIME DRESSING: 1 tbsp tamari soy sauce • **juice of 3 limes** • **1 tbsp xylitol** • **1 tsp deseeded and finely chopped red chilli** • **1 garlic clove, minced** • **1 tbsp chopped coriander leaves**

1 Mix together all the dressing ingredients in a bowl, then chill until needed.
2 Place the onion, mushrooms and pepper in a bowl and toss with the dressing. Leave for 10 minutes to soften. Add the rest of the ingredients and mix well.

HEALTH BENEFITS
*Kelp is rich in **minerals**, including **iodine**, plus **enzymes**, **potassium**, **magnesium**, **calcium**, **iron** and **amino acids**. It is also very **cleansing** and **detoxifying** for the body.*

Nutritional analysis per serving: *Calories 42kcal • Protein 2.1g • Carbohydrates 8.1g • Fat 0.5g (of which saturates 0.1g)*

caper tapenade-filled mushrooms >

Rich in flavour, chestnut mushrooms provide an earthy, meaty texture to this dish, but you could also use larger Portobello mushrooms. The longer you leave them in the dehydrator or oven, the softer they become. Mushrooms are also a source of protein, plus immune-boosting selenium, for raw fooders.

PREPARATION TIME: *15 minutes, plus 30 minutes marinating time* • **DEHYDRATING TIME:** *4 hours*
• **STORAGE:** *the tapenade can be prepared in advance and kept in the fridge for up to 3–4 days*
• **SERVES:** *4*

2 tbsp extra virgin olive oil • 1 tbsp balsamic vinegar • 12 chestnut mushrooms, or 4 Portobello mushrooms, stalks removed

CAPER TAPENADE: 100g/3½oz/heaped ¾ cup pitted green or black olives • 1 garlic clove, minced • 1 tbsp capers, rinsed • 2 tbsp basil leaves • 1 tbsp lemon juice • olive oil, to blend • 1 tomato, finely chopped

1 Drizzle the oil and the vinegar over the mushrooms and leave to marinate for 30 minutes while you make the tapenade.
2 To make the tapenade, place the olives, garlic, capers, basil and lemon juice in a blender and blend with enough oil to form a stiff paste. Mix in the tomato.
3 Spoon the tapenade on top of the mushrooms and place on a non-stick sheet placed on a baking or dehydrator tray. Put in a dehydrator set at 45°C/115°F, or place in an oven at 45°C/115°F (or on its lowest setting with the door ajar), for 4 hours.

HEALTH BENEFITS
*Rich in **vitamin E** and healthy **monounsaturated fats**, olives are a great addition to your raw week. Substituting **monounsaturated fat** for saturated fat in the diet has been shown to **aid weight loss** by enhancing the body's breakdown of fat, **improving insulin function** and keeping you **feeling fuller** for longer.*

Nutritional analysis per serving: *Calories 134kcal • Protein 0.7g • Carbohydrates 0.7g • Fat 14.1g (of which saturates 2.1g)*

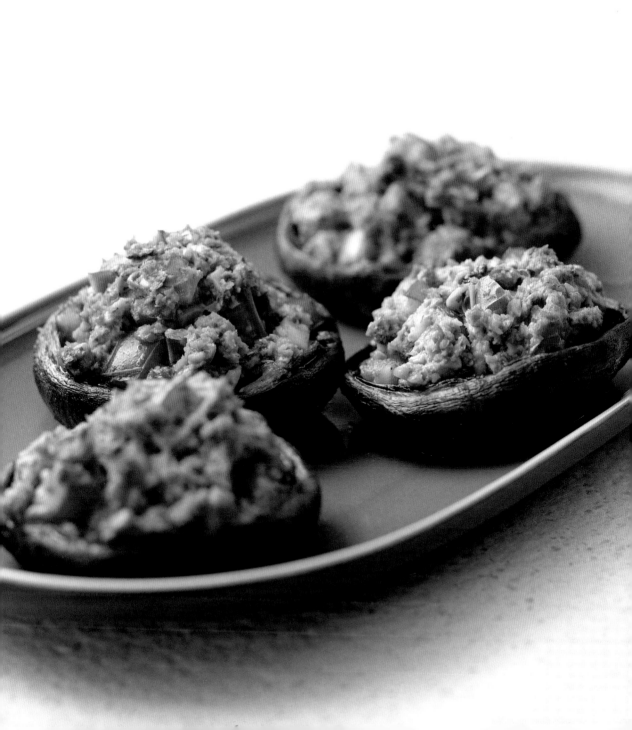

tamarind coconut curry with fig & apple chutney >

If you're craving a take-away, try this delicious raw curry instead. Using a combination of cauliflower, tomatoes and shiitake mushrooms creates a wonderful meaty texture to the dish.

PREPARATION TIME: *20 minutes* • **DEHYDRATING TIME:** *3 hours* • **STORAGE:** *will keep in the fridge for up to 2 days* • **SERVES:** *4*

1 small cauliflower, in tiny florets • 3 tomatoes, diced • 8 shiitake mushrooms, sliced • 2 tbsp olive oil • 2 tsp tamari • 1 tsp ground coriander • 1 tsp ground cumin

TAMARIND COCONUT SAUCE: 1 tsp tamarind paste • 30g/1oz/½ cup unsweetened, dried, shredded coconut flakes • ½ red pepper, deseeded • 2 tomatoes • 1 tsp xylitol • 2 tsp garam masala • 1 tbsp lemon juice • 1 large garlic clove • ½ tsp sea salt

FIG & APPLE CHUTNEY: 1 handful mint leaves, chopped • 1 green apple, cored and chopped • juice of ½ lime • ½ tsp sea salt • 150g/5½oz/1 cup chopped dried figs

1 Put all the ingredients for the curry in a bowl and mix together well. Put in a dehydrator set at 45°C/115°F, or place in an oven at 45°C/115°F (or on its lowest setting with the door ajar), for 2 hours.
2 To make the chutney, place all the ingredients in a food processor and pulse to form a chunky paste. Alternatively, just mix all the ingredients together in a bowl
3 To make the sauce, put all the ingredients in a blender and blend until smooth. Mix with the vegetables and return to the dehydrator or oven for 1 hour. Serve with the chutney.

HEALTH BENEFITS
*Tamarind is a source of **fibre**, as well as being rich in **antioxidants, vitamin C and many minerals**.*

Nutritional analysis per serving (with chutney): *Calories 252kcal • Protein 7g • Carbohydrates 30.4g • Fat 11.5g (of which saturates 1.4g)*

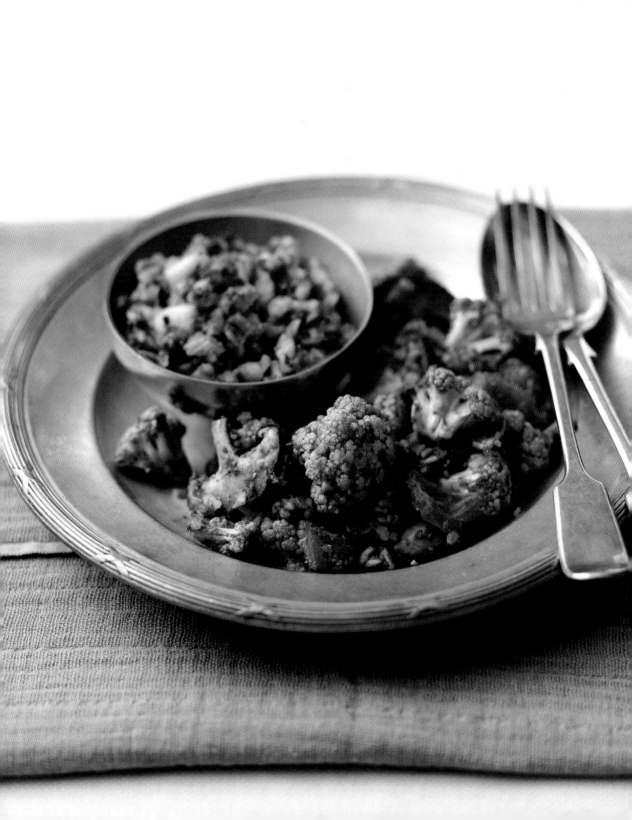

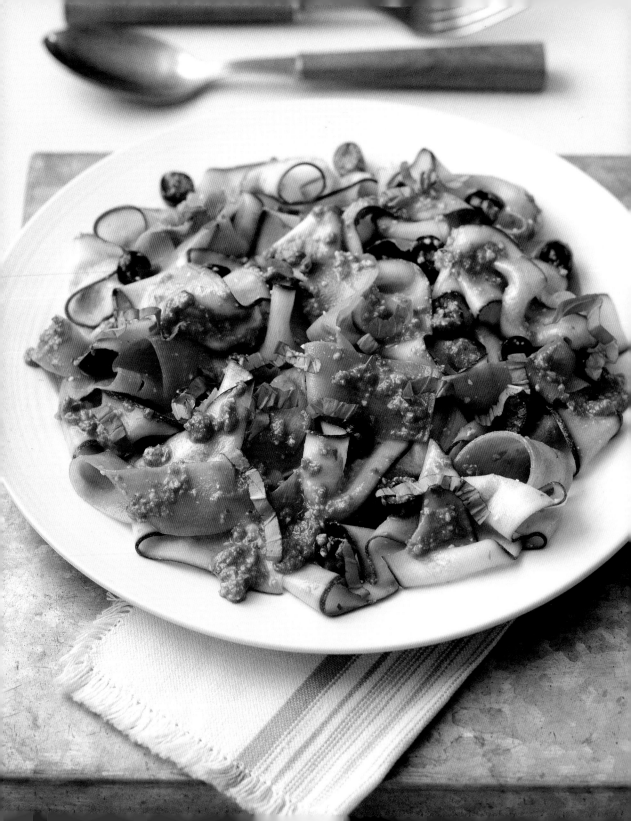

< vegetable pappardelle with red pepper & walnut sauce

A light "pasta" dish made from strips of carrot and courgette, and tossed with a creamy, red pepper sauce. Adding basil leaves and olives creates a wonderful simple Mediterranean low-carb dish. The sauce is equally delicious as a dip with vegetable sticks or crackers.

PREPARATION TIME: *20 minutes* • **STORAGE:** *the sauce will keep in the fridge for up to 2 days* • **SERVES:** *4*

2 courgettes • 2 carrots, peeled • pinch sea salt • 85g/3oz/⅔ cup pitted black olives, halved • 1 large handful basil leaves, shredded • freshly ground black pepper

RED PEPPER & WALNUT SAUCE: 1 tbsp tamari soy sauce • 1 garlic clove, minced • 1 red pepper, halved lengthways, deseeded and chopped • 6 sun-dried tomatoes, chopped • 30g/1oz/scant ¼ cup walnuts, chopped • 2 tbsp extra-virgin olive or walnut oil • 1 tbsp xylitol or yacon syrup • 1 tbsp lemon juice • 1 tsp sea salt

1 To make the sauce, place all the ingredients in a food processor and process until smooth. Add a little water to thin, if needed.
2 Using a swivel peeler, create long strips of courgette and carrot. Sprinkle with the salt. Place in a bowl with the black olives. Spoon over enough sauce to coat the vegetables and scatter over the basil leaves. Season with pepper to taste.

HEALTH BENEFITS
*Walnuts are a rich source of healthy **monounsaturated fats** and essential **omega-3 fatty acids**, plus **protein** and **fibre** – all important to support healthy weight loss. They are also rich in anti-inflammatory antioxidants, including **vitamin E, phenols, tannins and flavonoids**, and **melatonin** to help promote healthy sleep patterns.*

Nutritional analysis per serving: *Calories 214kcal • Protein 3g • Carbohydrates 8.6g • Fat 19.2g (of which saturates 2.6g)*

side dishes

mixed salad with caper, herb & citrus dressing >

A simple cleansing salad with a tangy, light dressing. The bitter leaves of chicory are mellowed by the sweet flavours of orange, beetroot and carrot.

PREPARATION TIME: *15 minutes* • **SERVES:** *4*

1 chicory head, sliced into 2cm/¾in pieces • 1 carrot, peeled and julienned • 1 raw beetroot, julienned • ½ red pepper, deseeded and julienned • 50g/2oz alfalfa sprouts (optional) • 225g/8oz mixed salad leaves, such as watercress, rocket and romaine lettuce • 2 spring onions, julienned

CAPER, HERB & CITRUS DRESSING: 2 tbsp capers, rinsed • 1 garlic clove, minced • 1 tbsp chopped parsley • 1 tsp white miso paste • 1 tbsp orange juice • 1 tbsp red wine vinegar • 2 tbsp extra virgin olive oil or flaxseed oil • ½ tsp sea salt • freshly ground black pepper

1 Place the chicory, carrot, beetroot and red pepper strips in a bowl with the alfalfa sprouts, if using, and the salad leaves. Scatter over the spring onions.
2 Mix together all the dressing ingredients in a bowl. Pour over the salad and serve immediately.

HEALTH BENEFITS
*Chicory and its relative endive are well-known **cleansing** and **digestive** aids, stimulating digestive enzymes and promoting the growth of **friendly bacteria in the gut**, which aids absorption of nutrients. They also include **terpenoids**, and other **phytonutrients**, which help cleanse the body and act as a mild diuretic to **reduce fluid retention**.*

Nutritional analysis per serving: *Calories 99kcal • Protein 2.4g • Carbohydrates 3.8g • Fat 8.4g (of which saturates 1.3g)*

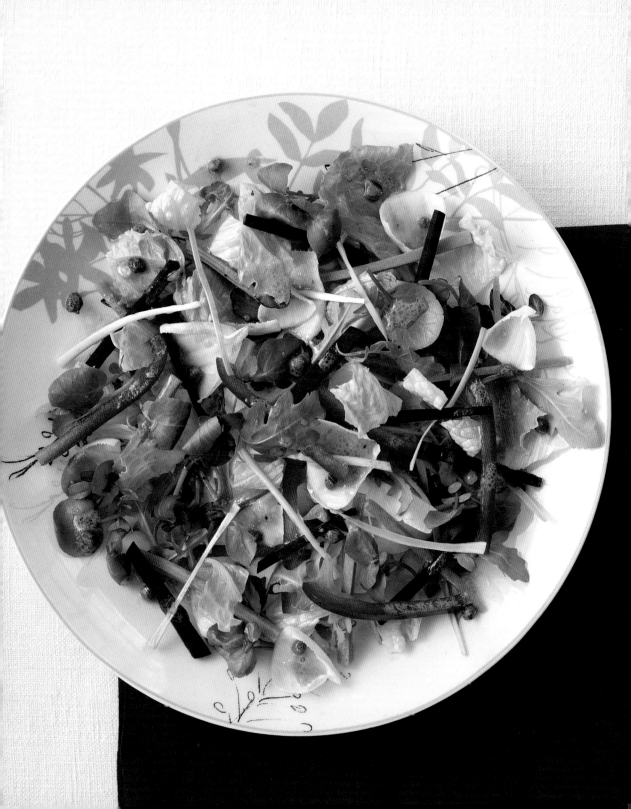

tomato & cider vinegar kale chips >

No raw food book is complete without a recipe for kale chips: a delicious low-calorie, nutrient-dense snack or accompaniment to a meal. This version combines creamy cashew nuts with sun-dried tomato and cider vinegar to form a tangy coating to the kale.

PREPARATION TIME: *15 minutes* • **DEHYDRATING TIME:** *8–10 hours or overnight* • **STORAGE:** *will keep in an airtight container for up to 2–3 days* • **SERVES:** *4*

450g/1lb kale, destalked and torn into pieces • 2 tbsp tamari soy sauce • 1 tomato, chopped • 4 tbsp apple cider vinegar • 1 tsp garlic salt • 4 pitted dates • 6 sun-dried tomatoes, chopped • ½ tsp smoked paprika • 1 tbsp cashew nut butter

1 Place the kale in a large bowl.
2 Place all the remaining ingredients in a blender and process until smooth. Add a little water to thin, if needed.
3 Pour the sauce over the kale and massage the marinade into the kale with your hands. Place the kale on mesh dehydrator trays and put in a dehydrator set at 45°C/115°F for 8–10 hours until crispy. Alternatively, place on baking trays and put in an oven at 45°C/115°F (or on its lowest setting with the door ajar) overnight.

HEALTH BENEFITS
Dried fruits, such as dates, add a wonderful sweetness to savoury dishes. They are rich in **soluble fibre** *to support* **elimination of waste** *and slow down the release of sugars into the body to* **keep energy levels high***.*

Nutritional analysis per serving: *Calories 109kcal • Protein 5.4g • Carbohydrates 6g • Fat 6.9g (of which saturates 0.8g)*

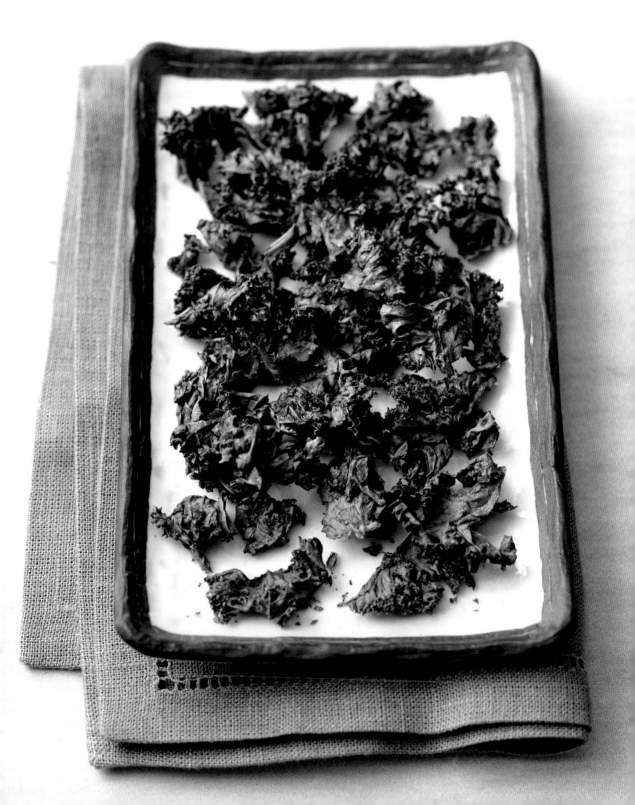

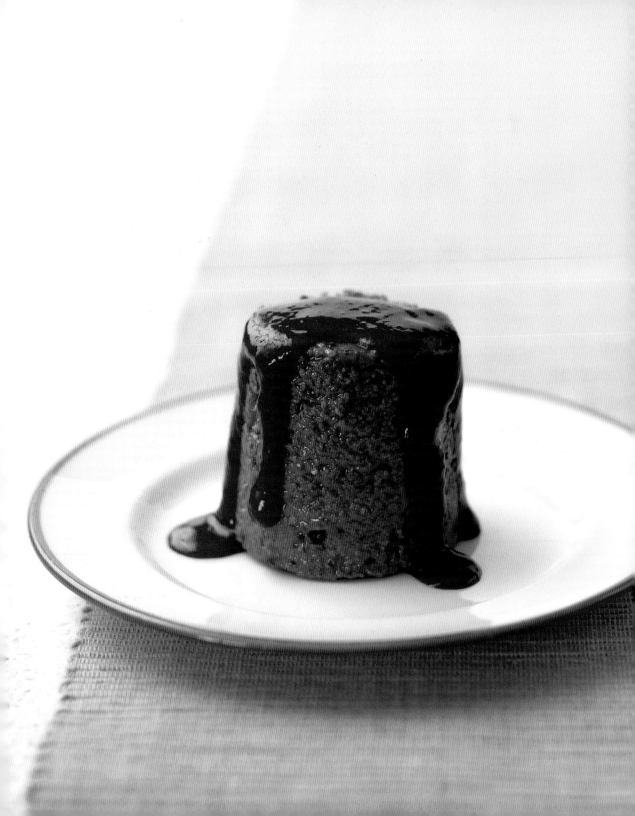

snacks

< cherry & raspberry ice

This easy-to-assemble "ice cream" does not require the use of an ice cream maker. I like to pour the mixture into individual non-stick pudding moulds or muffin cases, which I then turn out on to plates and drizzle with the sauce. You could use ramekins or other small freezer-proof pots instead to make these delicious low-sugar, protein-packed treats.

PREPARATION TIME: *15 minutes, plus 2–3 hours freezing time* • **STORAGE:** *the ice cream can be kept in the freezer for up to 3 days; the sauce can be kept in the refrigerator for up to 2 days* • **SERVES:** *6*

200g/7oz/1¼ cups macadamia nuts • 2 tsp vanilla extract • 60g/2¼oz/⅓ cup cherries, pitted • 60g/2¼oz/½ cup raspberries • 1 tbsp lemon juice • 4 tbsp xylitol or other sweetener • 125ml/4fl oz/½ cup pomegranate or cherry juice

RASPBERRY SAUCE: 100g/3½oz/heaped ¾ cup raspberries • 3 tbsp xylitol

1 To make the ice cream, place all the ingredients in a food processor and process until smooth. Pour into individual Teflon moulds or ramekins. Freeze for 2–3 hours.
2 To make the sauce, place the raspberries and xylitol in a blender and blend until smooth. Sieve for a smoother consistency, if you like.
3 Turn out the ices by running a knife around the inside of the moulds and dipping the moulds briefly in hot water. Drizzle over the sauce to serve.

HEALTH BENEFITS
*Raspberries, like other berries, are bursting with **vitamins** and **antioxidants** to help protect against the signs of **ageing** and **chronic disease**. They are particularly rich in **ellagic acid**, known for its **anti-cancer** properties, and soluble **fibre**, useful to help **curb appetite** and support **digestive health**.*

Nutritional analysis per serving: *Calories 312kcal • Protein 3.1g • Carbohydrates 23.5g • Fat 26g (of which saturates 3.8g)*

desserts

chocolate-orange hazelnut mousse >

A creamy, rich mousse, perfect for satisfying chocolate cravings. High in protein yet low in sugar, this is a great dessert for you to keep your blood sugar levels balanced while enjoying a delicious chocolate treat.

PREPARATION TIME: *10 minutes, plus 30 minutes chilling time* • **STORAGE:** *best eaten on the same day* • **SERVES:** *4*

2 avocados, halved, pitted and chopped • juice and zest of 2 oranges, plus extra to serve • 55g/2oz hazelnut butter • 35g/1¼oz/¼ cup hazelnuts • 50g/1¾oz/scant ½ cup raw cacao powder • 2 tbsp xylitol or other sweetener, to taste

1 Place all the ingredients in a food processor with 125ml/4fl oz/½ cup water and process until very smooth. Add a little extra water to thin, if needed.
2 Chill for 30 minutes before serving. Top with a little orange zest.

HEALTH BENEFITS
Oranges, like other citrus fruits, are known for their immune-boosting properties, being packed full of **bioflavonoids** *and* **vitamin C**, *which help stimulate the activity of white blood cells. A good source of* **soluble fibre**, *including* **pectin, essential oils and citric acid**, *they are also wonderful cleansers, helping to* **absorb fats and toxins** *from the digestive tract.*

Nutritional analysis per serving: *Calories 326kcal • Protein 7.1g • Carbohydrates 21.3g • Fat 24.5g (of which saturates 3.6g)*

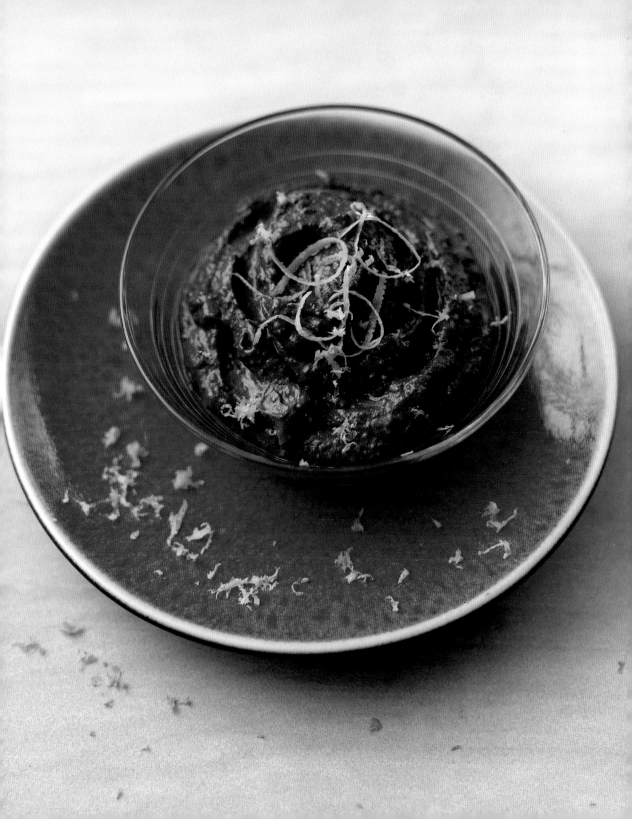

flower pollen & green tea ice >

This refreshing, instant ice cream is made by using frozen sliced bananas and cashew nut milk to create a creamy, low-calorie treat. This is also a delicious way to sneak more greens into your diet. The addition of green tea boosts the antioxidant profile and has been shown to stimulate metabolism, so assisting weight loss.

PREPARATION TIME: *10 minutes + 4 hours or overnight freezing time* • **STORAGE:** *will keep in the freezer for up to 1 month* • **SERVES:** *4*

---

4 small bananas, sliced • 125g/4½oz/heaped ¾ cup cashew nuts • 2 tbsp plus 1½ tsp flower pollen • 10g/¼oz/¼ cup baby spinach leaves • 1 tsp vanilla extract • 2 tbsp matcha green tea powder

1 Place the bananas in a lidded container and freeze for 4 hours or overnight.
2 Place the cashew nuts, pollen, spinach, vanilla extract, green tea powder and 250ml/ 9fl oz/1 cup water into a food processor and process until smooth.
3 Add the bananas and process again until creamy and smooth. Serve immediately or spoon into a shallow freezer-proof container and freeze. Take out of the freezer 20 minutes before serving to soften slightly.

HEALTH BENEFITS
*A complete superfood, flower pollen is **nourishing** and **energizing**, containing an incredible array of **vitamins, minerals, amino acids and enzymes**. It is thought to help weight loss by stimulating metabolism, helping emulsify fats and reducing cravings. It is especially rich in **B vitamins and antioxidants**, including **lycopene, selenium, beta-carotene, vitamin C, vitamin E**, as well as many **flavonoids**.*

Nutritional analysis per serving: *Calories 283kcal • Protein 8.7g • Carbohydrates 26.2g • Fat 15.7g (of which saturates 3.1g)*

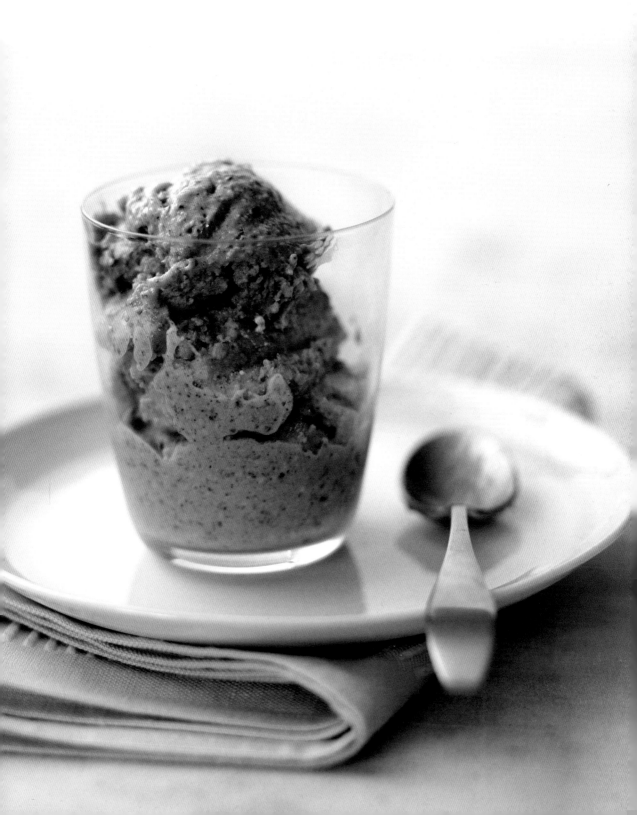

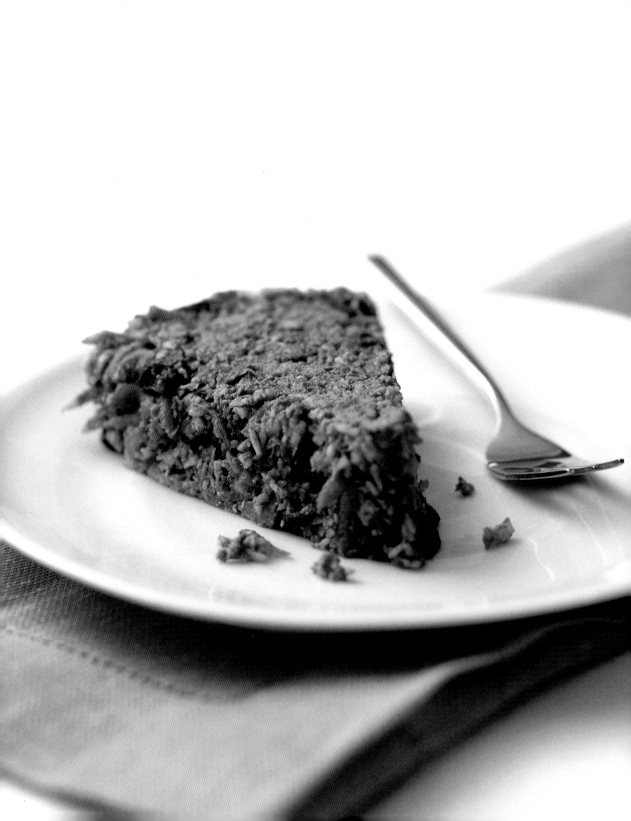

< toffee apple & carrot cake

This light, raw cake uses mesquite and raw cacao to create a delicious toffee-caramel flavour. Instead of using a large cake tin, you could press the mixture into individual ring moulds. You can dehydrate the mixture for a couple of hours in a dehydrator or cool oven to create a drier texture.

SOAKING TIME: *15 minutes* • **PREPARATION TIME:** *20 minutes, plus 2–3 hours chilling time* • **STORAGE:** *will keep in the fridge for up to 3 days* • **MAKES**: *10–12 portions*

2 apples, peeled, cored and finely grated • 2 carrots, peeled and finely grated • 115g/4oz/scant 1¼ cups pecans, finely ground • 80g/2¾oz/scant 1 cup desiccated coconut • 2 tbsp mesquite powder • 2 tbsp raw cacao powder • ½ tsp cinnamon • pinch sea salt • 150g/5½oz/scant 1¼ cups raisins • 60g/2¼oz/½ cup dried apple (soaked for 15 minutes, then drained) • 60g/2¼oz/⅓ cup pitted dates (soaked for 15 minutes, then drained) • 1 whole orange, peeled

1 Place the apples and carrots in a large bowl with the pecans, coconut, mesquite powder, cacao powder, cinnamon, salt and raisins.
2 Place the dried apple and dates in a blender with the orange. Process to form a paste. Add to the nut mixture and combine thoroughly. Place the mixture in batches in a food processor and pulse to form a wet dough. Do not over-mix.
3 Press the mixture into a greased and baking parchment-lined 20cm/8in round cake tin and chill for 2–3 hours before serving in slices.

HEALTH BENEFITS
*Mesquite meal is a traditional Native American food that is high in **protein** and rich in minerals, including **calcium, magnesium, potassium, iron and zinc**. It has a sweet, rich, molasses-like flavour with a hint of caramel, which blends well into smoothies or other drinks, especially those made with cacao and maca.*

Nutritional analysis per serving: *Calories 168kcal • Protein 2.3g • Carbohydrates 19.9g • Fat 8.7g (of which saturates 0.7g)*

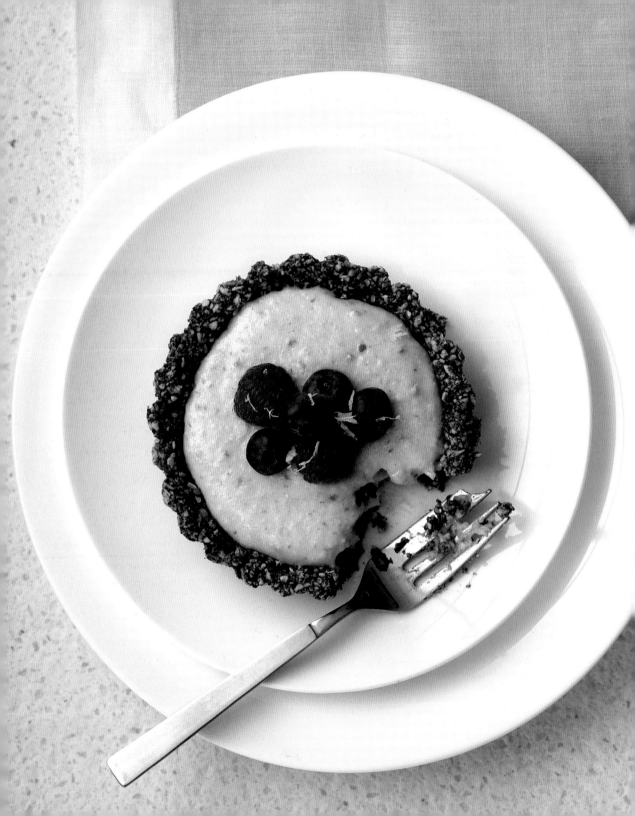

< acai berry tarts with lemon custard

These mini tarts can be prepared in advance and kept frozen until needed. Adding banana to the filling reduces the calorie content, while the cashew nuts provide plenty of protein to provide a satisfying, filling treat.

PREPARATION TIME: *20 minutes, plus 4 hours or overnight freezing time* • **STORAGE:** *will keep in the fridge for up to 1 day. Can be frozen for up to 1 month* • **MAKES:** *4 individual tarts*

CRUST: 175g/6oz/heaped 1 cup cashew nuts • 40g/1½oz/scant ½ cup desiccated coconut • 2 tbsp acai powder • 1 tsp sea salt • 60g/2¼oz/⅓ cup pitted dates • juice and zest of 1 lemon

FILLING: 1 large banana, sliced • juice and zest of 2 lemons • 2 tbsp xylitol or other sweetener • 60g/2¼oz/⅓ cup pitted dates • 60g/2¼oz/heaped ⅓ cup cashew nuts • 1 tsp sea salt • fresh berries, to serve • grated lemon zest, to serve

1 Put the banana in a lidded container and freeze for 4 hours or overnight.
2 To make the crust, place the cashew nuts and coconut in a food processor and process until fine. Mix in the acai powder and salt. Blend the dates and lemon juice and zest in a blender to form a paste, then mix into the nuts to form a dough. Press into four greased mini tart tins and freeze for 1 hour. Remove from the tins before filling.
3 To make the filling, blend the lemon juice and zest, xylitol and dates in a blender to form a thick paste. Add the remaining ingredients and blend to form a creamy custard. Spoon into the tart cases and decorate with the fresh berries and lemon zest.

HEALTH BENEFITS
*Acai berries are a wonderful superfood, exceptionally rich in **antioxidants**, particularly **anthocyanins** and **flavonoids**, which help reduce the **signs of ageing** and protect against **chronic disease**. They contain plenty of **B vitamins** for combating stress and maintaining energy, and also **calcium**, **potassium and magnesium**. Dried acai powder is particularly **high in fibre** to support the cleansing of toxins and elimination of waste, plus **protein** and **omega-3 fatty acids** to support weight loss.*

Nutritional analysis per tart: *Calories 541kcal • Protein 12.2g • Carbohydrates 41.8g • Fat 35.6g (of which saturates 9.6g)*

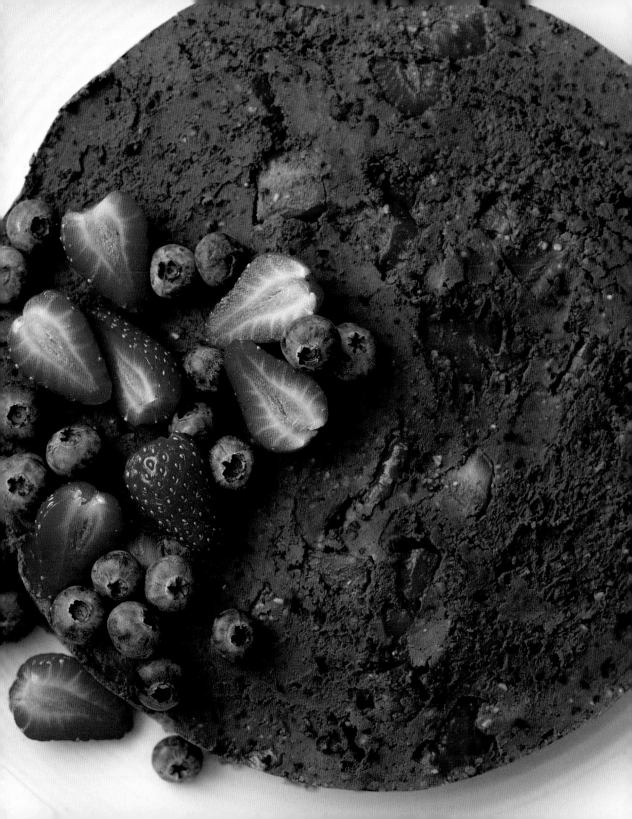

CHAPTER 3

The Raw for Life Diet

If you've enjoyed the benefits of the Raw Food Weekend or the Raw Food Week and want to experience more radiant energy and a youthful, lean body longer term, it's time to increase your intake of raw foods for life.

That does not have to mean 100% raw. Many people experience renewed health and wellbeing while eating a moderate amount of cooked food alongside raw food dishes. However, for great long-lasting health, try to include a range of raw foods in your diet daily.

In this chapter you will find two examples of a 100% raw menu, but feel free to mix and match with healthy cooked foods. There is no need to run out of ideas or feel deprived with raw food. Enjoy a wonderful array of smoothies, raw cereals, wraps, marinated foods, raw burgers and a delicious range of scrummy, indulgent raw puddings, cakes and treats, suitable for all the family.

< mixed berry chocolate torte (page 150)

the raw for life programme

Building up your intake of raw food slowly and gradually is the most sustainable way to move to a high raw food diet. Initially aim for one raw meal each day using any of the recipes in this book.

Often people find a raw breakfast or lunch and a green juice or smoothie the easiest way to start. You could then include a raw soup as part of the evening meal. Ideally, aim for around half of your diet to be raw, with the emphasis on healthy, nutrient-dense foods – quality rather than quantity is the focus. Many people experience renewed health and well-being while eating raw food dishes alongside a moderate amount of cooked food. But for maximum benefit, make sure your cooked food is as healthy as possible – whole foods, ideally organic and minimally processed without added sugars and trans fats. Avoid processed foods such as white flour, sugar, rice and other refined carbohydrates, ready meals and fast foods. Fried foods, caffeine, alcohol and sugary drinks should also be restricted. You should also make sure your body is fully hydrated, so drink plenty of pure water, herbal teas, juices and smoothies throughout the day. Make sure you eat plenty of vegetables (particularly leafy greens) rather than excessive fruit and raw desserts. Try to have a green juice or smoothie daily, and keep sweeteners of any type to a minimum. Eat a variety of different foods to give yourself the broadest spectrum of nutrients.

For optimum nutrition, a high raw diet should focus around the following foods:

• Sprouted seeds, beans and grains
• Leafy greens and other raw vegetables
• Fresh, ripe fruits, with the focus on low glycemic fruit such as berries, apples, pears, plums and apricots
• Sea vegetables
• Fermented foods such as sauerkraut and kimchi
• Smoothies, juices, raw soups, coconut water and water
• Nut and seed oils, olive oil, coconut butter, nuts, seeds and avocados

raw for life sample days

day one

On waking Large glass of hot water with juice of ½ lemon

Breakfast Watermelon Strawberry Crush (**page 120**), Sweet Papaya Chia Delight (**page 121**)

Lunch Curried Butternut Squash & Apple Soup (**page 124**), Flaxseed Crackers (**page 28**), raw salad

Snack Choc Chip Apricot Cookie Bar (**page 148**)

Dinner Teriyaki "Stir Fry" (**page 144**), Passionfruit & Orange Cheesecake (**page 154**)

day two

On waking Cup of herbal/peppermint tea

Breakfast Choc-Cinnamon Crunchies (**page 121**) with nut milk and fresh berries

Lunch Tropical Salad with Miso Dressing (**page 126**) and Moroccan Beetroot Dip (**page 129**)

Snack Berry Shake (**page 120**)

Dinner Caramelized Onion Tart with Nut Cheese, Tomatoes & Olives, leafy green salad (**page 140**), Mixed Berry Chocolate Torte (**page 151**)

If you are eating animal or fish protein, make sure it is organic/free-range/grass-fed/wild-caught for maximum health benefits. If you suffer from digestive health problems, you may wish to try simple food combining. Key rules are: avoid drinking with meals as this dilutes digestive juices; eat fruit separately; and keep concentrated protein away from starchy carbohydrates.

To get you started on a high raw diet, I have suggested two sample days using some additional recipes for you to enjoy. You will notice that this chapter includes a few extra fruit dishes, which are useful for an occasional treat or for entertaining friends or family. While the suggested meal plan focuses on raw foods, you may wish to include some cooked food, or warm through a raw soup or raw dish.

breakfasts

watermelon strawberry crush

A wonderfully refreshing drink, bursting with vitamin C and beta-carotene, yet low in calories. Add the watermelon seeds when blending as they provide antioxidant-rich vitamin E.

PREPARATION TIME: *10 minutes* • STORAGE: *best drunk immediately, but will keep in the fridge for up to 1 day.* • SERVES: *2*

350g/12oz watermelon, deseeded and cubed • 12 strawberries • zest of 1 lime • 1 mint leaf

1 Place all the ingredients in a blender and blend until smooth. Serve chilled.

HEALTH BENEFITS
*Watermelon is rich in **beta-carotene** and **lycopene**. A great source of **potassium**, it can help maintain **body fluid balance**, making it great for tackling **bloating** and **water retention**.*

Nutritional analysis per serving: *Calories 74kcal • Protein 1.5g • Carbohydrates 15.6g • Fat 0.6g (of which saturates 0.2g)*

berry shake

This potent combination of superfoods will keep your body energized.

SOAKING TIME: *15 minutes* • PREPARATION TIME: *15 minutes + 4 hours freezing time* • STORAGE: *best drunk immediately* • SERVES: *4*

1 banana • 250g/9oz/1⅔ cups strawberries • 60g/2¼oz/½ cup goji berries (soaked in 250ml/9fl oz/1 cup water for 15 minutes) • 2 tsp shelled hemp seeds • 500ml/17fl oz/2 cups coconut water • 2 tsp lucuma powder • 2 tbsp xylitol or flower pollen • 2 tsp cashew nut butter • 1 tsp flaxseed oil

1 Put the banana in a lidded container and freeze for 4 hours or overnight.
2 Blend all the ingredients, including the soaking liquid, together until smooth.

HEALTH BENEFITS
*Antioxidant-rich strawberries are rich in **ellagic acid, anthocyanidins and phenols**, known to help **fight disease** and protect against **free-radical damage**.*

Nutritional analysis per serving: *Calories 165kcal • Protein 3.9g • Carbohydrates 31.2g • Fat 3.9g (of which saturates 0.2g)*

sweet papaya chia delight

A healthy breakfast treat that also makes a great snack or dessert.

PREPARATION TIME: *30 minutes* • **STORAGE:** *will keep in the fridge for up to 2 days* • **SERVES:** *4*

40g/1½oz/¼ cup chia seeds • 20g/¾oz/ scant ¼ cup desiccated coconut • 40g/1½oz/¼ cup cashew nuts • 2 sharon fruit, chopped • 1 papaya, deseeded and chopped • 2 tsp lucuma powder • pulp of 2 passionfruit • unsweetened coconut flakes, to serve

1 Mix the chia seeds and coconut.
2 Blend the remaining ingredients, except the passionfruit, plus 250ml/9fl oz/1 cup water until smooth and creamy. Pour it over the chia seed mixture and leave for 20 minutes, stirring occasionally as it thickens.
3 Spoon into bowls. Drizzle over the fruit pulp and scatter with coconut flakes.

HEALTH BENEFITS
*Papaya is great for **immune health**. It also contains **papain** – perfect for **detoxifying**.*

Nutritional analysis per serving: *Calories 183kcal • Protein 5.1g • Carbohydrates 15.3g • Fat 11.8g (of which saturates 4.3g)*

choc-cinnamon crunchies

Mix with chopped nuts and dried fruit as a tasty trail mix, or use as a cereal.

SOAKING TIME: *overnight* • **PREPARATION TIME:** *10 minutes* • **DEHYDRATING TIME:** *6 hours* • **STORAGE:** *once completely dry, will keep in an airtight container for up to 1 week* • **SERVES:** *4*

100g/3½oz/¾ cup buckwheat groats (soaked overnight) • 1 tsp cinnamon • 2 tsp raw cacao powder • 1 tbsp coconut butter, melted (see page 17) • 1 tsp yacon syrup (optional) • chopped nuts, to serve • fresh fruit, to serve • Almond Milk or Chocolate Milk, to serve (see page 24)

1 Rinse and drain the buckwheat and add the cinnamon, cacao, coconut butter and yacon syrup, if using. Mix well.
2 Dehydrate for 6 hours until crispy, following the instructions on page 68.
3 Mix with chopped nuts and fruit, and pour nut milk over to serve.

HEALTH BENEFITS
*Buckwheat is rich in **manganese, magnesium and flavonoids**, especially rutin.*

Nutritional analysis per serving: *Calories 137kcal • Protein 2.5g • Carbohydrates 22.2g • Fat 4.4g (of which saturates 3.4g)*

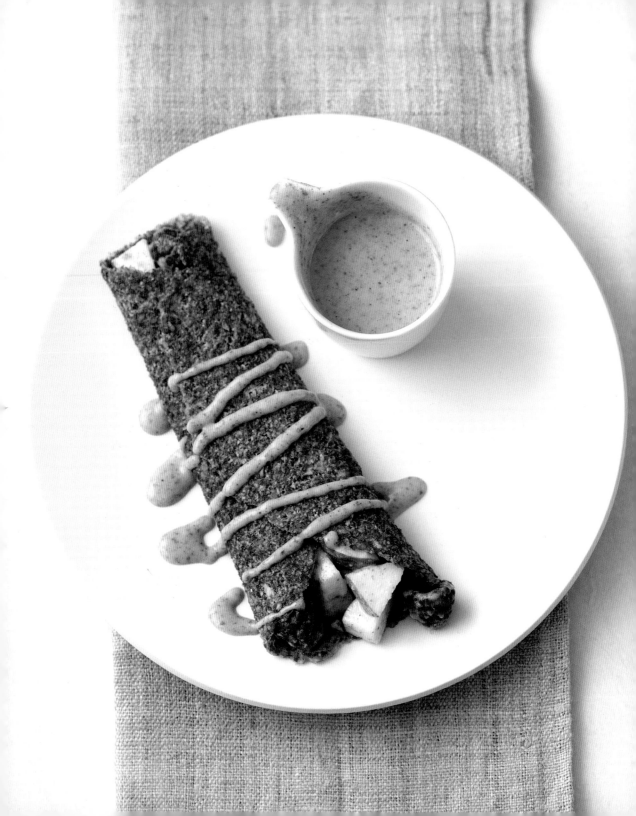

< apple crêpes with caramel sauce

Deliciously light crêpes, which can be rolled up with a fruit filling and served drizzled with a healthy caramel sauce packed with superfoods.

PREPARATION TIME: *20 minutes* • **DEHYDRATING TIME:** *2–3 hours* • **STORAGE:** *the sauce will keep in the fridge for up to 2 days. The crêpes will keep in an airtight container for up to 1 day* • **SERVES:** *4*

2 apples, diced • 40g/1½oz/½ cup ground flaxseeds • 4 pitted dates • 150g/5½oz fruit, such as berries and chopped apple or pear, to serve

CARAMEL SAUCE: 100g/3½oz almond butter • 2 tbsp xylitol or yacon syrup • 1 tsp lucuma powder • 1 tsp mesquite powder • 1 tsp maca root powder • pinch ground cinnamon • pinch sea salt • 60g/2¼oz/⅓ cup dates • 1 tsp vanilla extract

1 To make the crêpes, place the diced apples, flaxseeds and dates in a blender with 125ml/4fl oz/½ cup water and blend until smooth.
2 Spread the mixture into 4 thin circles on a Teflon non-stick sheet placed on a baking or dehydrator tray. Put in a dehydrator set at 45°C/115°F for 2–3 hours until dry but still flexible. Alternatively, place in an oven at 45°C/115°F (or on its lowest setting with the door ajar), though this may take a little longer.
3 To make the sauce, place all the ingredients and 185ml/6fl oz/¾ cup water in a blender and process until smooth. Add a little more water for a thinner sauce.
4 Mix a little of the sauce with the berries and chopped fruit and spoon inside each crêpe. Roll up and drizzle over the remaining sauce.

HEALTH BENEFITS
*Lucuma is a **nutrient-dense** fruit from Peru that tastes like butterscotch. A natural sweetener used in ice cream and smoothies, it also supplies plenty of **beta-carotene, niacin (B3), calcium and iron**.*

Nutritional analysis per serving: *Calories 285kcal • Protein 8.1g • Carbohydrates 33g • Fat 16.1g (of which saturates 0.8g)*

lunches

curried butternut squash & apple soup >

A warming autumn soup, naturally sweet and lightly spiced, that will help with weight loss. The creaminess of the squash avoids the need to add nuts or seeds to the soup, keeping this light and refreshing. Top with a few spiced seeds to serve.

PREPARATION TIME: *20 minutes* • **STORAGE:** *will keep in the fridge for up to 2 days* • **SERVES:** *4–6*

1 large butternut squash, deseeded and diced • juice of 2 oranges • 2 tomatoes • 2 apples, diced • 2 tsp garam masala • freshly ground black pepper • 4 pitted dates, chopped • pinch sea salt • Spiced Seeds (see page 29), to sprinkle

1 Place the butternut squash and orange juice into a food processor and process to form a paste.
2 Add the remaining ingredients and 500ml/17fl oz/2 cups warm water and continue to process until blended. Warm in a large bowl in a dehydrator or cool oven for 20 minutes, if you like.
3 Spoon the soup into bowls and sprinkle with the spiced seeds to serve.

HEALTH BENEFITS
A delicious starchy vegetable, butternut squash is rich in **soluble fibre**, *making it a fantastic aid to* **digestive health**. *It also provides a wealth of* **antioxidants** *for optimal health, including* **beta-carotene, lutein and zeaxanthin**, *which are particularly beneficial for eye health.*

Nutritional analysis per serving (for 4): *Calories 119kcal • Protein 3.1g • Carbohydrates • 20.7g • Fat 2.5g (of which saturates 0.3g)*

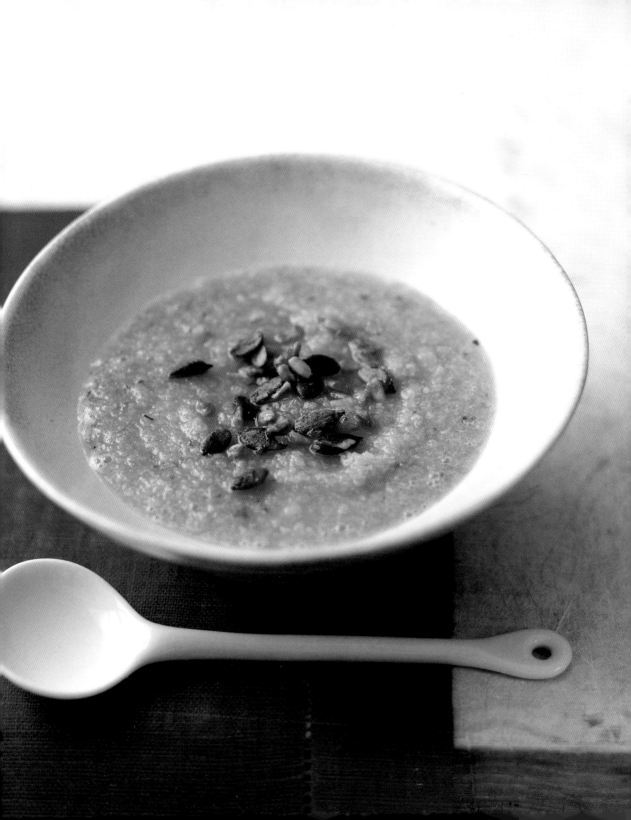

tropical salad with miso dressing >

This refreshing salad is perfect for summer. The combination of the salty miso and tangy lime juice creates a fabulous dressing that would also work well with sea vegetables. The tamari-coated cashew nuts add some tasty crunch.

PREPARATION TIME: *15 minutes* • **DEHYDRATING TIME:** *4–6 hours* • **STORAGE:** *will keep in the fridge for up to 2 days* • **SERVES:** *4*

60g/2oz/heaped ⅓ cup cashew nuts • 2 tbsp tamari soy sauce • 1 cucumber, cut into 5cm/2in lengths, then julienned • 6 lychees, peeled, pitted and quartered • 1 small ripe mango, sliced • 225g/8oz mixed rocket and watercress leaves • handful coriander leaves • 1 red chilli, deseeded and finely chopped

MISO DRESSING: 1 tbsp white miso paste • 3 tbsp flaxseed oil • juice of 1 lime • 1 tbsp xylitol

1 Place the cashew nuts and tamari in a bowl and mix to coat. Spread the nuts on a non-stick sheet placed on a dehydrator tray. Put in a dehydrator set at 45°C/115°F for 4–6 hours, turning them over as they dry. Alternatively, place in an oven at 45°C/115°F (or on its lowest setting with the door ajar) for 6 hours.
2 Place the cucumber in a bowl with the fruit, salad leaves, coriander and chilli.
3 To make the dressing, whisk all the ingredients together in a jug or bowl. Drizzle over the salad and toss to coat. Sprinkle with the cashew nuts, to serve.

HEALTH BENEFITS
*Sweet and juicy lychees are a wonderful, healthy tropical fruit. A good source of **vitamin C** and **polyphenols**, they can be beneficial for supporting **immune function**. They are also a useful source of **B vitamins**, needed for energy production, plus **potassium** to help prevent fluid retention.*

Nutritional analysis per serving: *Calories 259kcal • Protein 6g • Carbohydrates 16.7g • Fat 19.4g (of which saturates 2.6g)*

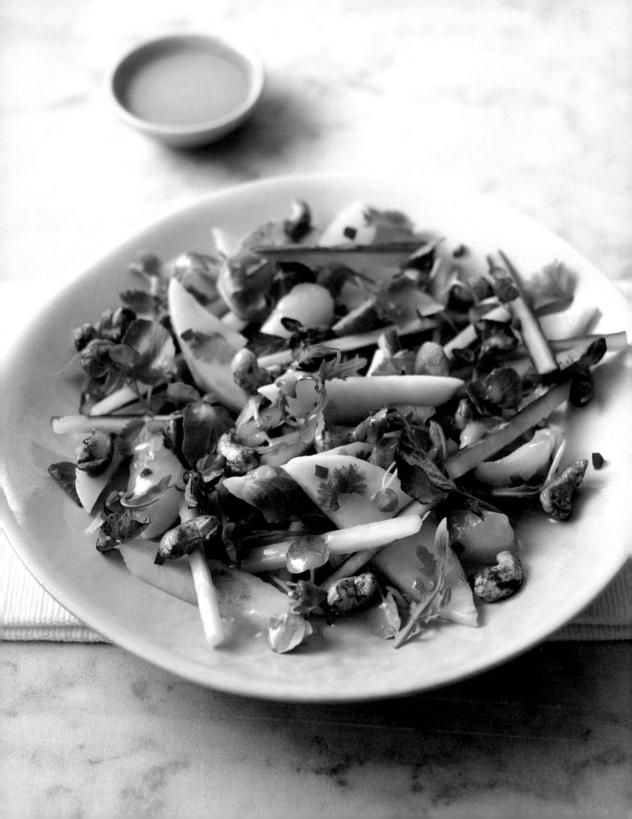

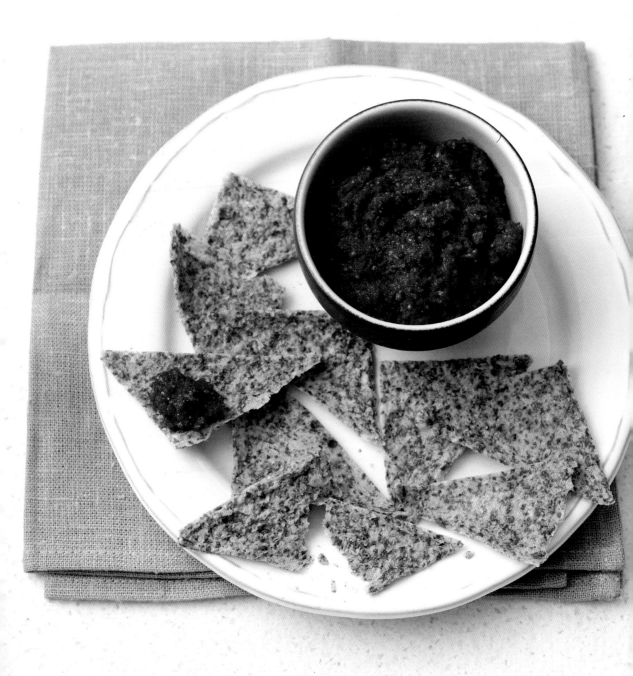

< moroccan beetroot dip

This creamy, lightly spiced, vibrant purple dip makes a perfect speedy light meal or snack served with Corn Chips (see page 31), or Flaxseed Crackers (see page 28), and a selection of vegetable sticks. Packed with protein, it will help to curb your appetite while keeping you energized throughout the day.

PREPARATION TIME: *15 minutes* • **STORAGE**: *will keep in the fridge for up to 3–4 days*

125g/4½oz/heaped ¾ cup cashew nuts • ½ tsp ground cumin • ½ tsp ground coriander • pinch paprika • 1 raw beetroot, peeled and chopped • 2 tsp lemon juice • ½ tsp sea salt

1 Place all the ingredients in a blender and blend until well mixed, adding a little water to thin, as necessary.
2 Transfer to a bowl and serve with corn chips or flaxseed crackers.

HEALTH BENEFITS

*A well-known **detoxifier** and **blood cleanser**, beetroot also contains a wealth of nutrients to boost **immune function** and keep you **energized**. The combination of **iron and folic acid** helps build **red blood cells**, preventing fatigue, while its natural sugars and fibre provide lasting **energy**. Bursting with powerful **antioxidants**, including **beta-cyanin**, which can help improve the function of **detoxification** enzymes in the **liver**, it can also support **kidney health** by increasing bile production, which is needed for **emulsifying fats** in the body.*

Nutritional analysis per tablespoon: *Calories 57kcal • Protein 1.8g • Carbohydrates 2g • Fat 1.7g (of which saturates 0.9g)*

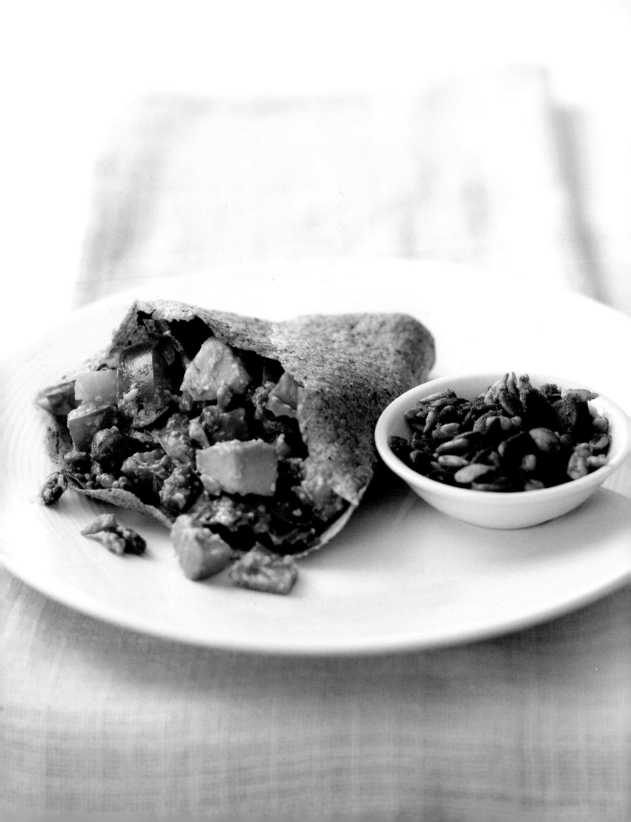

< caesar wraps

A raw version of the classic salad is used to fill Courgette Wraps (see page 31). As an alternative, use romaine lettuce leaves or cabbage leaves to keep these wraps light and low carb, yet substantial enough for a light lunch.

PREPARATION TIME: *15 minutes* ● **STORAGE:** *the dressing will keep in the fridge for up to 3–4 days. The wraps are best eaten immediately once assembled* ● **SERVES:** *6*

6 Courgette Wraps (see page 31) ● 3 tbsp Sweet Caesar Dressing (see page 26) ● 6 tbsp Spiced Seeds (see page 29)

FILLING: 1 small head romaine lettuce, chopped ● 1 avocado, halved, pitted and diced ● 3 tbsp capers, drained and rinsed ● 2 tomatoes, deseeded and diced ● 1 tbsp dried nutritional yeast flakes

1 Combine all the filling ingredients in a large bowl. Lightly coat one side of each wrap with a little dressing.
2 Place a spoonful of the salad along the bottom third of one of the wraps and roll up to enclose. Repeat with the remaining wraps and serve immediately.

HEALTH BENEFITS
*Romaine lettuce is a highly nutritious salad leaf, yet low in calories and wonderfully hydrating. It is rich in **antioxidants**, including **vitamin C and beta-carotene**, and contains energizing **B vitamins**, and the minerals **chromium, magnesium and potassium**.*

Nutritional analysis per serving: *Calories 215kcal ● Protein 6g ● Carbohydrates 8.7g ● Fat 18g (of which saturates 1.6g)*

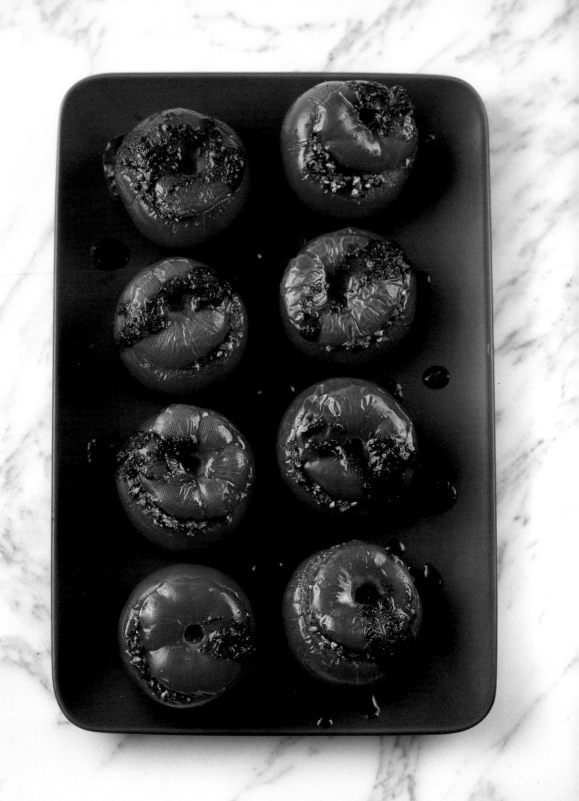

< semi-dried tomato cups with pistachio pesto and basil oil

A simple, summery dish filled with a light raw pesto, and packed with anti-aging and immune-boosting ingredients. Perfect as a lunch or light evening meal accompanied with a Caesar salad or simple green salad.

PREPARATION TIME: *20 minutes* • **DEHYDRATING TIME:** *4 hours* • **STORAGE:** *the basil oil will keep in the fridge for up to 1 week* • **SERVES:** *4*

8 vine-ripened tomatoes • 1 garlic clove, minced • 1 tbsp extra virgin olive oil • freshly ground black pepper • 8 tbsp Pistachio Pesto (see page 88)

BASIL OIL: 30g/1oz/1 cup basil leaves • 4 tbsp extra virgin olive oil • pinch sea salt

1 To make the basil oil, place the ingredients in a blender and blend until smooth, then sieve. Store in a squeezy bottle in the fridge until needed.
2 Cut a small lid off the top of each tomato, and with a teaspoon carefully remove the pulp and seeds. If necessary, cut a small piece off the base of each tomato to ensure it stands upright. Place on a non-stick sheet on a baking or dehydrator tray.
3 Mix the garlic with the oil and drizzle into the tomatoes. Season with pepper and replace the lids. Put in a dehydrator set at 45°C/115°F, or place in an oven at 45°C/115°F (or on its lowest setting with the door ajar), for 3 hours to soften.
4 Fill the tomatoes with the pesto, replace the lids and return to the dehydrator or oven for 1 hour to warm through. Drizzle with a little of the basil oil to serve.

HEALTH BENEFITS
Tomatoes are a great source of immune-supporting **antioxidants**, *including* **vitamin C and E, beta-carotene and zinc**. *They are packed with* **lycopene**, *which may protect against* **heart disease** *and certain* **cancers**. *Being rich in* **vitamin K**, *they also help support* **bone health**. *A wonderfully hydrating fruit, they aid* **weight loss and healthy digestion**.

Nutritional analysis per serving: *Calories 293kcal • Protein 4.2g • Carbohydrates 6.1g • Fat 28.1g (of which saturates 4g)*

dinners

courgette & spinach lasagne >

Strips of courgette replace traditional pasta in this dish, which is dressed with a sweet tomato sauce and a creamy nut cheese sauce. Chopped olives have been included in this recipe for extra texture. Make this the day before serving to allow the flavours to develop.

PREPARATION TIME: *45 minutes* • **DEHYDRATING TIME:** *1 hour* • **STORAGE:** *will keep in the fridge for up to 2 days* • **SERVES:** *6*

3 courgettes • 1 tbsp olive oil, plus extra to drizzle • sea salt, to sprinkle • 175g/6oz/ 1¾ cups mixed green and black pitted olives, finely chopped • 2 garlic cloves, minced • 1 tbsp chopped basil leaves • 1 recipe quantity Basic Nut Cheese (see page 25) • 1 recipe quantity Sun-dried Tomato Sauce (see page 27) • 55g/2oz/2 cups baby spinach leaves • freshly ground black pepper

1 Thinly slice the courgettes lengthways with a swivel peeler or mandolin. Drizzle over a little oil and a sprinkling of salt and leave to soften for 15 minutes.
2 Mix together the olives, garlic, basil and 1 tbsp olive oil in a bowl. To assemble, place one-third of the courgette strips in the base of a rectangular or square baking dish, overlapping the strips slightly. Spread over half the nut cheese, then half the tomato sauce, and dot with half the olive mixture. Top with half the spinach leaves. Repeat the layering, finishing with a final layer of courgette strips. Season the top with pepper.
3 Warm through in a dehydrator or cool oven for 1 hour before serving, if you like.

HEALTH BENEFITS
*Leafy greens like spinach are an essential part of any raw food diet. Perfect for **tackling fatigue**, spinach is packed with **iron, vitamin C and folic acid** for **healthy blood cells**. It is also rich in **chlorophyll**, a wonderful **energizer**, and an effective **cleanser** and **detoxifier** to support liver health.*

Nutritional analysis per serving: *Calories 404kcal • Protein 9.6g • Carbohydrates 12.4g • Fat 35.2g (of which saturates 5.6g)*

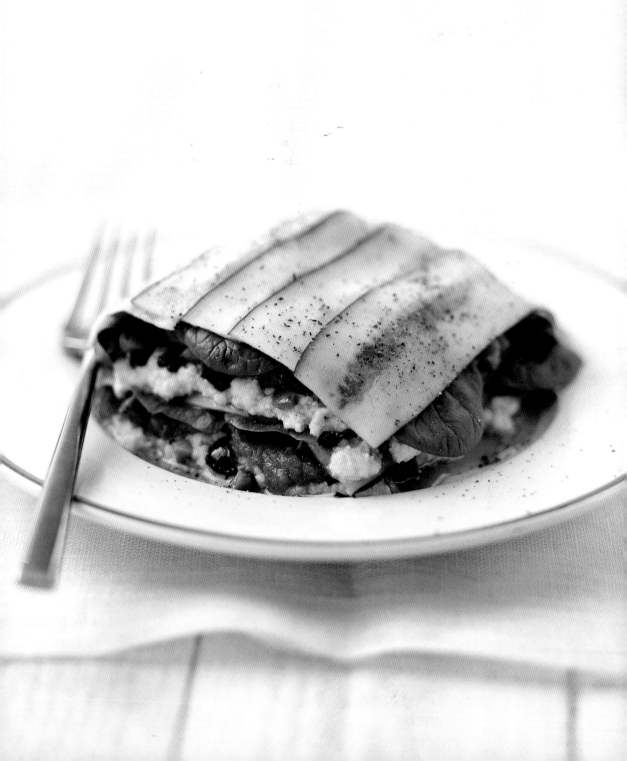

coriander falafel with tahini cream >

A meaty-style recipe, delicious served with the tahini cream. Serve with a large mixed salad or wrap in a Tortilla or Courgette Wrap (see page 31).

SOAKING TIME: *30 minutes* • **PREPARATION TIME:** *20 minutes* • **DEHYDRATING TIME:** *8 hours or overnight* • **STORAGE:** *will keep in the fridge for up to 2 days* • **SERVES:** *4*

60g/2¼oz/½ cup sunflower seeds • 60g/2¼oz/⅓ cup pumpkin seeds • 2 tbsp coriander leaves • ½ tsp ground cumin • ½ tsp ground coriander • 6 sun-dried tomatoes, soaked for 30 minutes and chopped • 1 garlic clove, minced • 1 shallot, finely chopped • 60g/2¼oz/½ cup pitted green or black olives, chopped • pinch smoked paprika • ½ tsp sea salt • 1 handful mixed salad leaves, to serve

TAHINI CREAM: 3 tbsp tahini • 2 tsp xylitol • 2 tbsp lemon juice • pinch sea salt

1 Place all the falafel ingredients in a food processor and process until completely mixed. Shape into walnut-sized balls and place directly on a mesh dehydrator sheet or a baking sheet. Put in a dehydrator set at 45°C/115°F, or place in an oven at 45°C/115°F (or on its lowest setting with the door ajar), for 8 hours or overnight until firm.
2 To make the tahini cream, place all the ingredients in a blender with 2 tbsp water and blend until smooth and creamy. To serve, place the salad leaves on a platter, top with the falafel and drizzle over the cream.

HEALTH BENEFITS

*Pumpkin seeds are a rich source of **B vitamins** and **minerals**, including **zinc, iron, copper and manganese** to support **energy levels** and **immune health**. A useful source of **protein**, they help to **curb appetite** and **stabilise blood sugar levels**, and have **omega-3 fats** to support **metabolism**.*

Nutritional analysis per serving: *Calories 301kcal • Protein 9.2g • Carbohydrates 8g • Fat 26.1g (of which saturates 3.7g)*

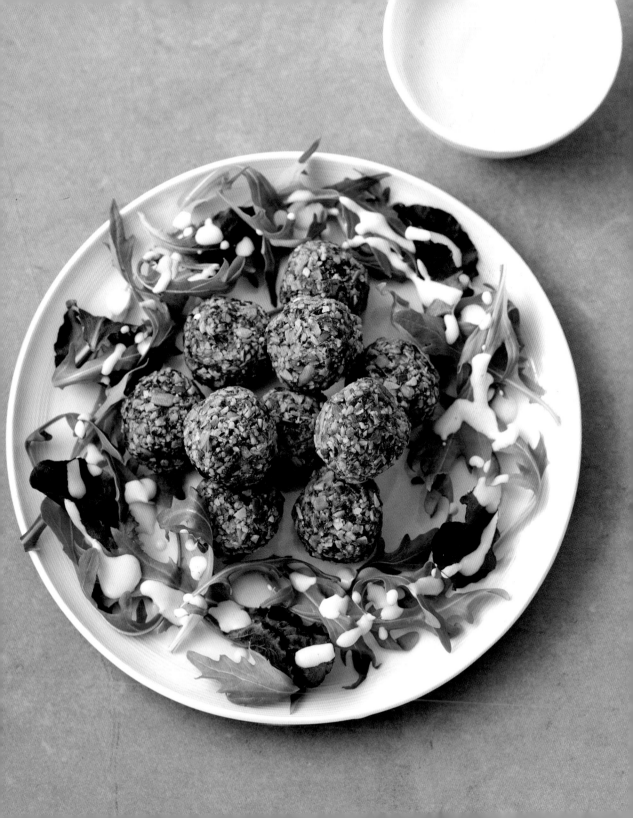

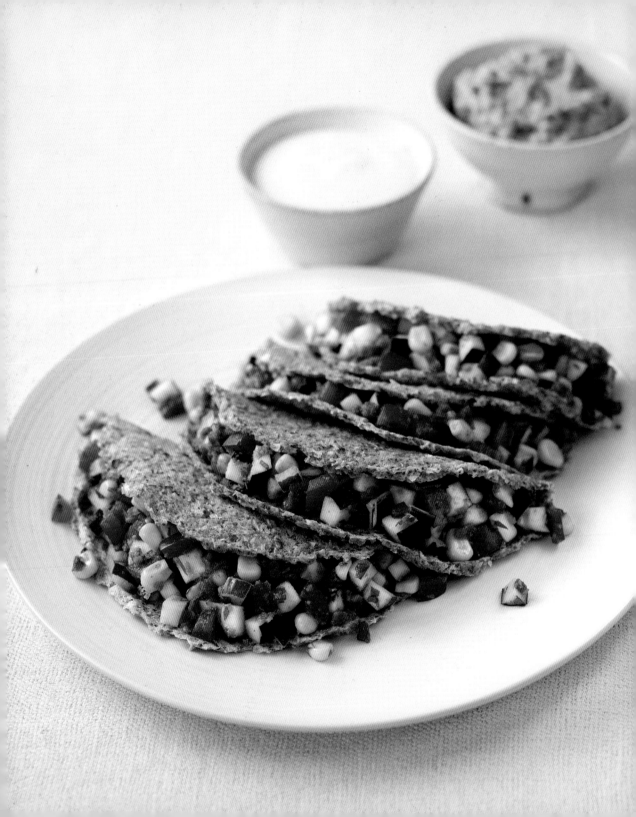

< spicy enchiladas with guacamole

Enchiladas are a popular dish. Here they are made with raw tortillas and filled with a chunky sweetcorn salsa and topped with a rich tomato sauce. In addition to the guacamole, serve Lime Sour Cream (see page 80), if wanted.

PREPARATION TIME: *30 minutes* • **DEHYDRATING TIME:** *1 hour* • **STORAGE:** *chill the guacamole in the fridge for up to 1 day before using* • **SERVES:** *4*

---

4 Tortillas (see page 31)

FILLING: 1 courgette, finely diced • ½ red onion, finely diced • 60g/2¼oz/heaped ⅓ cup sweetcorn (scraped off the cob or frozen) • 115g/4oz mixed sprouted beans and seeds (optional) • 1 red pepper, halved lengthways, deseeded and chopped • 1 red chilli, deseeded and chopped • 1 tbsp chopped coriander leaves • 1 recipe quantity Sun-dried Tomato Sauce (see page 27)

GUACAMOLE: 1 large ripe tomato, finely chopped • 2 large ripe avocados, halved, pitted, and flesh spooned out • juice of 1 lime • handful coriander leaves, roughly chopped • ½ red onion, finely chopped • ½ tsp sea salt • 1 red chilli, deseeded and finely chopped

1 To make the guacamole, place all the ingredients in a food processor. Pulse lightly to combine. Spoon into a bowl, cover with cling film and chill until needed.
2 Place all the filling ingredients except the tomato sauce in a bowl. Add enough sauce to coat lightly. Put in a dehydrator set at 45°C/115°F, or place in an oven at 45°C/115°F (or on its lowest setting with the door ajar), for 1 hour to warm through.
3 Spoon the mixture on to the tortillas, gently fold over and serve with the guacamole.

HEALTH BENEFITS
Packed with **phytonutrients** *and* **volatile oils**, *coriander is well known for its antimicrobial properties, making it useful for tackling* **digestive upsets**.

Nutritional analysis per serving (with guacamole): Calories 403kcal • Protein 7g • Carbohydrates 26.1g • Fat 30.2g (of which saturates 4.4g)

caramelized onion tart with nut cheese, tomatoes & olives >

This delicious tart combines a creamy nut cheese with tangy balsamic onions, sweet tomatoes and salty olives. Warm through in a cool oven or dehydrator before serving and accompany with a simple green salad.

PREPARATION TIME: *40 minutes* • **DEHYDRATING TIME:** *11½ hours* • **STORAGE:** *will keep in the fridge for up to 2 days* • **SERVES:** *4–6*

1 tart crust (see page 93) • 2 tbsp olive oil • 60g/2¼oz/⅓ cup pitted dates • 2 tbsp tamari soy sauce • 2 tbsp balsamic vinegar • 2 large red onions, thinly sliced • 8 cherry tomatoes, halved • 60g/2¼oz/½ cup pitted black olives, chopped • 3 tbsp Basic Nut Cheese (see page 25) • 4 basil sprigs • freshly ground black pepper

1 Press the tart crust into a greased round 20cm/8in tart or pie dish and put in a dehydrator set at 45°C/115°F, or place in an oven at 45°C/115°F or on its lowest setting with the door ajar), for 8 hours or overnight.
2 Place the oil, dates, tamari and vinegar in a food processor and blend to form a paste. Add 4 tbsp water to form a thick sauce. Coat the onions in the sauce and place on a non-stick sheet placed on a baking or dehydrator tray. Season with pepper and dehydrate for 3 hours until soft, at the same temperature as used above.
3 Scatter the onions, tomatoes and olives in the tart case and drop spoonfuls of the cheese over them. Warm through in a dehydrator or cool oven for 30 minutes, then scatter with the basil leaves before serving.

HEALTH BENEFITS
*Basil is well known for its **anti-microbial** effects, being rich in oils that help **reduce inflammation** and kill **harmful bacteria**. A great source of **antioxidants**, it is also excellent for promoting **cardiovascular health** and protecting against the **signs of ageing**.*

Nutritional analysis per serving (for 4): *Calories 446kcal • Protein 10.3g • Carbohydrates 19.5g • Fat 37g (of which saturates 12.7g)*

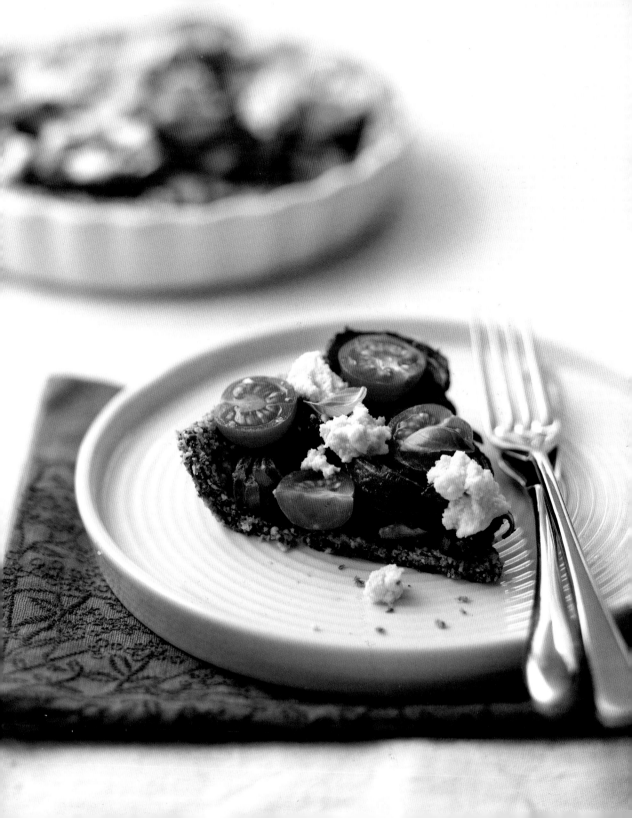

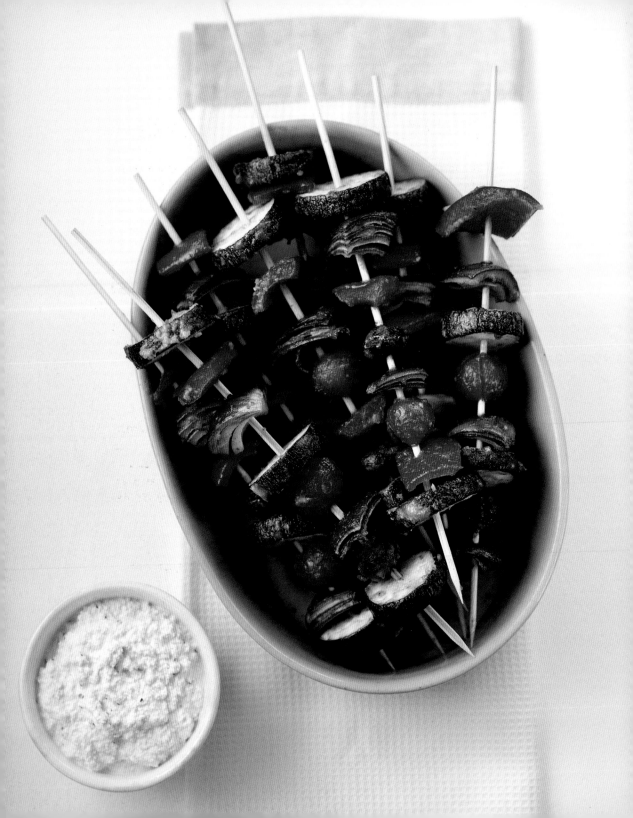

< marinated mediterranean vegetables with harissa cheese

A simple, prepare-ahead dish that requires minimum effort but is packed full of flavour. Marinate the vegetables for an hour before dehydrating in a dehydrator or oven. Serve on skewers for a barbecue-style dish.

PREPARATION TIME: *30 minutes, plus 1 hour marinating time* • **DEHYDRATING TIME:** *2 hours*
• **SERVES:** *4*

1 courgette, cut into 1cm/½in slices • 1 red pepper, halved lengthways, deseeded and cut into chunks • 8 cherry tomatoes • 8 button mushrooms • 1 red onion, cut into chunks • 8 tbsp Harissa Cheese (see page 25), to serve

MARINADE: ½ red chilli, deseeded and chopped • 1 plum tomato, chopped • 1 garlic clove, minced • 1 spring onion, chopped • 4 pitted dates • ½ tsp sea salt • pinch paprika • 4 tbsp extra virgin olive oil

1 Place the vegetables in a shallow dish. Place the marinade ingredients in a blender and process until smooth. Pour over the vegetables, coat well and marinate for 1 hour.
2 Thread the vegetables on to skewers and place on a non-stick sheet placed on a baking or dehydrator tray. Put in a dehydrator set at 45°C/115°F, or place in an oven at 45°C/115°F (or on its lowest setting with the door ajar), for 2 hours. Serve with the harissa cheese, adding a little more water if needed to form a thick sauce.

HEALTH BENEFITS
*Red peppers are loaded with protective, immune-supporting nutrients, particularly **lycopene, beta-carotene and vitamin C**. They also contain **flavonoids**, which are thought to enhance the activity of **vitamin C** and protect the body against disease. Red peppers are a good source of **fibre**, which is needed to support **elimination of waste** and maintain **healthy digestive function**.*

Nutritional analysis per serving: *Calories 271kcal • Protein 3.5g • Carbohydrates 7.4g • Fat 25.4g (of which saturates 2.9g)*

teriyaki "stir fry" >

An easy-to-assemble, raw "stir fry", coated in a light, Asian-style, tangy sauce, combining tart vinegar, spicy ginger and garlic, and a little sweetness from the yacon syrup. Perfect for those occasions when you don't want to spend ages in the kitchen. Letting the vegetables marinate helps to soften them, creating a "cooked" texture. You can also dehydrate them for a couple of hours, if you like. For a more substantial meal, add a handful of kelp noodles before serving.

PREPARATION TIME: *15 minutes, plus 2 hours marinating time* • **DEHYDRATING TIME:** *2 hours (optional)* • **SERVES:** *4*

---

1 small pak choi, sliced • 85g/3oz mangetout • 6 shiitake mushrooms, sliced • 1 carrot, peeled and julienned • ½ red pepper, deseeded and julienned • 1 spring onion, julienned • 2 slices of pineapple, cut into chunks • 1 handful bean sprouts (optional)

DRESSING: 4 tbsp tamari soy sauce • 2 tbsp extra virgin olive oil • 2 tbsp pineapple juice • 1 tsp toasted sesame oil • 3 tbsp yacon syrup, to taste • 1 tsp grated ginger • 1 garlic clove, minced • 1 tsp onion powder

1 Mix together all the dressing ingredients in a bowl.
2 Place the vegetables and pineapple in a large bowl and pour over the dressing ingredients. Leave to marinate for 2 hours.
3 Put in a dehydrator set at 45°C/115°F, or place in an oven at 45°C/115°F (or on its lowest setting with the door ajar), for 2 hours before serving, if you like.

HEALTH BENEFITS
*Pak choi is a delicious Asian leafy green vegetable rich in **B vitamins**, including **B6** and **folate** to help keep you **energized and alert** throughout the day. Like other members of the cabbage family, it is rich in protective **phytonutrients**, including antioxidants **beta-carotene and vitamin C**.*

Nutritional analysis per serving: *Calories 156kcal • Protein 3.6g • Carbohydrates 18.2g • Fat 9.6g (of which saturates 1.3g)*

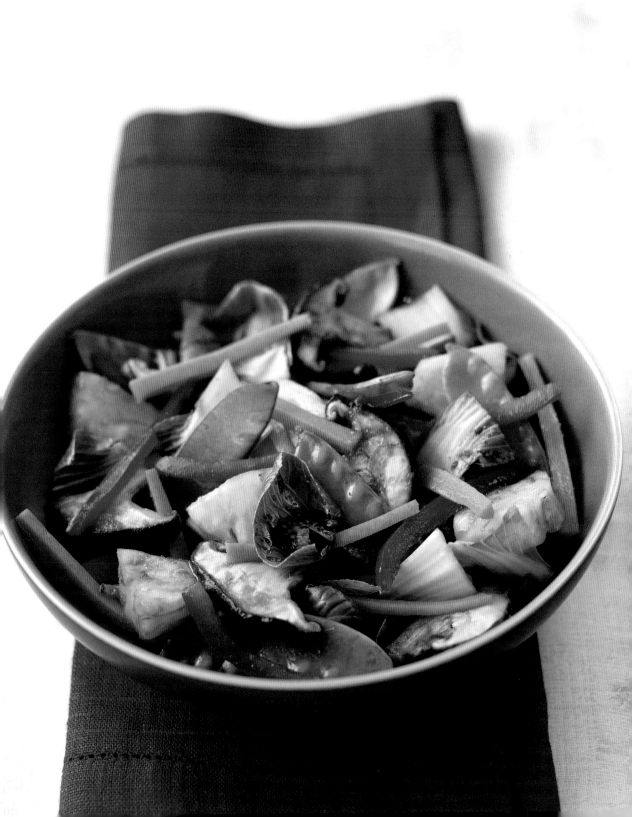

side dishes

speedy kale salad >

Kale is incredibly alkalinizing and packed full of nutrients. The kale leaves soften and wilt when mixed with the dressing ingredients, giving it a "cooked" texture, so allow it to sit for at least 10 minutes before serving.

PREPARATION TIME: *10 minutes, plus 10 minutes resting time* • **STORAGE:** *will keep in the fridge for up to 2 days* • **SERVES:** *4–6*

500g/1lb 2oz kale leaves • 2 tsp garlic salt • 300g/10½oz/2 cups cherry tomatoes, halved • 4 shiitake mushrooms, sliced • 2 tbsp mixed seeds

DRESSING: 2 ripe avocados, halved, pitted and flesh spooned out • 2 tsp tamari soy sauce • ½ tsp onion powder • pinch smoked paprika • 2 tbsp flaxseed oil • 2 tsp xylitol • juice of ½ lemon

1 Wash the kale and remove any tough stalks. Chop into small pieces and place in a large bowl.
2 Massage the garlic salt into the kale, squeezing the leaves until they begin to wilt. Add the remaining salad ingredients to the kale.
3 Place the dressing ingredients in a blender and blend until smooth.
4 Pour the dressing over the kale and massage into the salad using your hands. Allow to rest for 10 minutes before serving.

HEALTH BENEFITS
*Kale is a nutritional powerhouse, packed full of **phytochemicals, protein, vitamins and minerals**. It is a rich source of **glucosinolates**, known for their **anti-cancer properties**, plus **flavonoids and carotenoids**, including **beta-carotene, lutein and zeaxanthin**. A great bone booster too: full of **vitamin K**, which, along with **calcium and magnesium**, promotes strong **healthy bones**. A superb **cleansing** vegetable, it packs a nutritional punch and is perfect for supporting **weight loss**.*

Nutritional analysis per serving: *Calories 181kcal • Protein 5g • Carbohydrates 5.9g • Fat 15.6g (of which saturates 2.6g)*

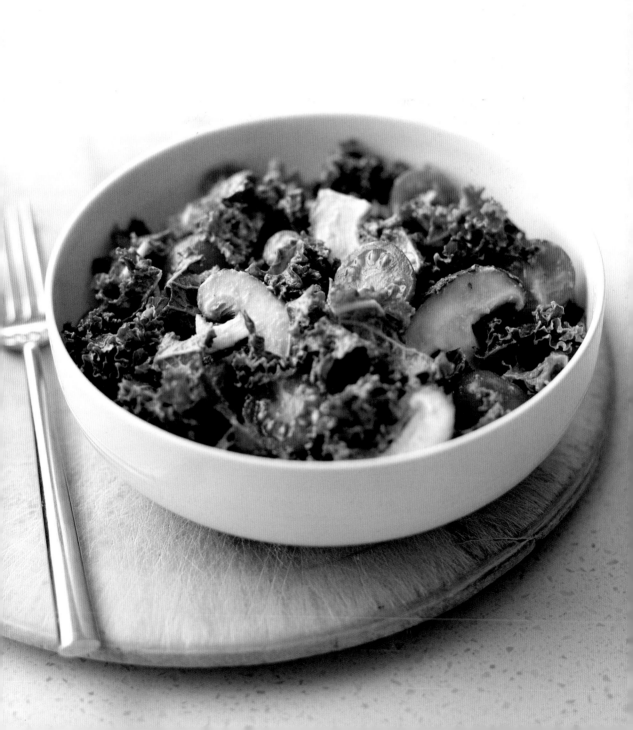

snacks

choc chip apricot cookie bars >

These delicious, chewy cookie bars are great to grab and go, making a nutritious breakfast option when time is tight. Being high in protein and sweetened naturally with dried fruit, they won't upset blood sugar levels either.

PREPARATION TIME: *20 minutes* • **DEHYDRATING TIME:** *8–10 hours* • **STORAGE:** *will keep in an airtight container in the fridge for up to 3–4 days* • **MAKES:** *12 cookie bars*

115g/4oz/scant 1¼ cups pecans • 2 tbsp whole flaxseeds • 125g/4½oz/heaped ¾ cup cashew nuts • pinch cinnamon • 2 tbsp raw cacao powder • pinch sea salt • 175g/ 6oz/scant 1 cup dried, ready-to-eat apricots, chopped • 4 tbsp raw cacao nibs

1 Place the pecans and flaxseeds in a blender and blend until finely chopped. Repeat with the cashew nuts, allowing some of the nuts to remain coarsely chopped for texture. Place in a bowl. Add the cinnamon, cacao powder and salt.
2 Place the apricots in a food processor and process to form a thick purée, then add to the nut mixture to form a dough. Stir in the cacao nibs.
3 Spread the mixture into a rectangle about 1cm/⅜in thick on a non-stick sheet placed on a baking or dehydrator tray. Mark into bars and put in a dehydrator set at 45°C/115°F, or place in an oven at 45°C/115°F (or on its lowest setting with the door ajar), for 6 hours. Flip over and dry for another 2–4 hours. The mixture should still be chewy. Alternatively, press the mixture into a shallow tin lined with cling film, then mark into bars. Freeze until firm (3–4 hours), then move to the fridge for 1 hour before eating.

HEALTH BENEFITS
*If you suffer from dips in energy levels, add cinnamon to your food. Cinnamon is a well-known spice for **stabilizing blood sugar levels**, **improving insulin function** and **fat burning**.*

Nutritional analysis per bar: *Calories 196kcal • Protein 4.9g • Carbohydrates 11.2g • Fat 15.3g (of which saturates 3g)*

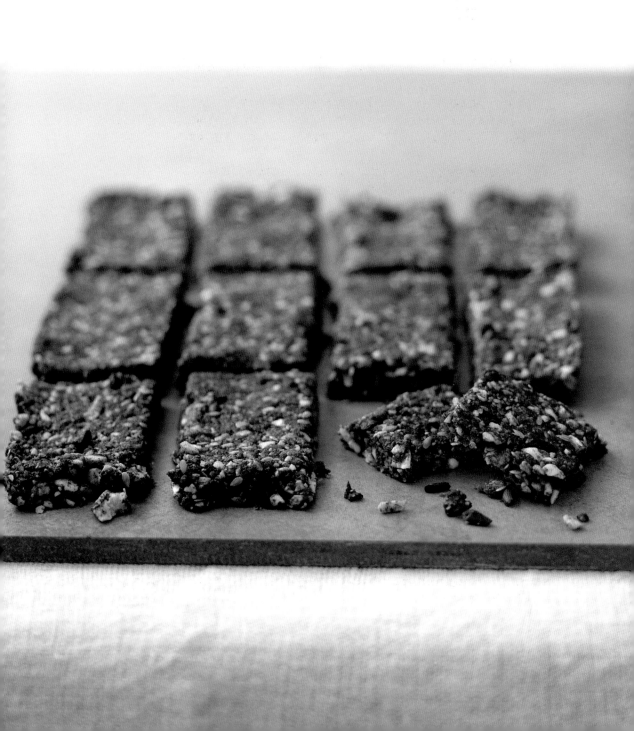

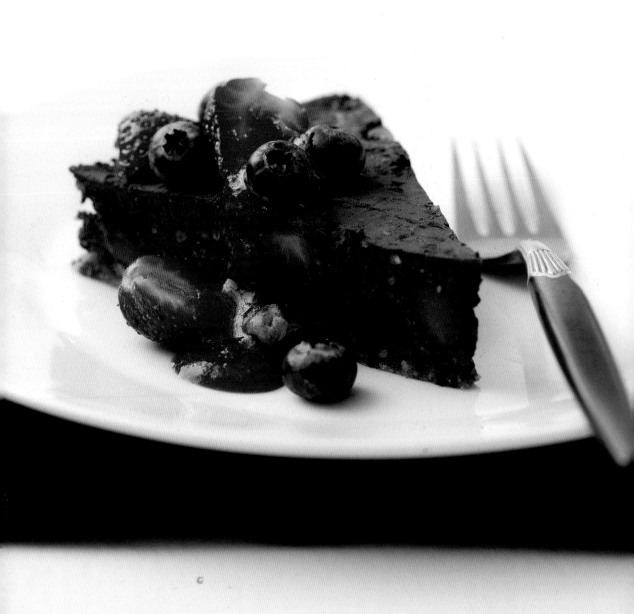

desserts

< mixed berry chocolate torte

Perfect for entertaining or when you want to treat yourself. You can also freeze the torte and serve it as an iced dessert. Accompany with mixed summer berries and a berry sauce, if you like.

SOAKING TIME: *15 minutes* • **PREPARATION TIME:** *30 minutes, plus 2–3 hours chilling time* • **STORAGE:** *will keep in the fridge for up to 3–4 days. Will freeze for up to 1 month* • **SERVES:** *10–12*

150g/5½oz/1½ cups pecans • grated zest of 1 lemon • 85g/3oz/scant ½ cup pitted dates (soaked for 15 minutes, then drained) • 3 tbsp melted coconut butter (see page 17) • 70g/2½oz/scant ½ cup cashew nuts • 50g/1¾oz/heaped ⅓ cup raw cacao powder • 115g/4oz cacao butter, grated and melted (see page 17) • 2 tbsp xylitol or other sweetener • juice of 1 lemon • 150g/5½oz/1 cup blueberries • 150g/5½oz/1 cup strawberries, chopped

1 Place the pecans in a blender and blend until finely chopped. Place in a bowl with the lemon zest. Place the dates in the blender with the coconut butter and blend to form a purée. Stir into the pecans to form a dough. Press into a 20cm/8in springform cake tin and chill.
2 Place the cashew nuts, cacao powder, cacao butter, xylitol, lemon juice and blueberries in a food processor and process until smooth. Fold in the strawberries.
3 Spread over the crust and chill for 2–3 hours until set.

HEALTH BENEFITS
*Blueberries are bursting with powerful **anti-ageing, immune-supporting and disease-protecting antioxidants**, including **anthocyanidins, vitamins C and E, selenium and zinc**. Rich in **pectin**, a type of soluble fibre, blueberries are a great cleanser, promoting the **elimination of toxins** and supporting **digestive health**. They have been shown to **reduce abdominal fat, lower cholesterol and improve insulin sensitivity** – great for maintaining a healthy weight.*

Nutritional analysis per serving (for 10, without serving suggestions): *Calories 280kcal • Protein 3.4g • Carbohydrates 12.7g • Fat 24.7g (of which saturates 9.9g)*

sharon fruit & mango sorbet >

A light, low-calorie dessert full of tropical flavours and naturally sweet, avoiding the need to add any sweetener. Use bags of frozen mango chunks to make a speedy sweet treat. Make sure the sharon fruit are very ripe so that they blend easily.

PREPARATION TIME: *15 minutes* • **FREEZING TIME:** *3–4 hours* • **SERVES:** *4*

2 ripe sharon fruit, chopped • 125ml/4fl oz/½ cup orange juice • 1 large mango, pitted and chopped, then frozen for 3–4 hours

1 Place the sharon fruit and orange juice in a blender and blend until smooth.
2 Add the frozen mango chunks and process on high to create a soft, creamy ice.
3 Serve immediately or spoon into a shallow, freezer-proof container and freeze until required. Take it out of the freezer 15 minutes before serving, to soften slightly.

HEALTH BENEFITS
Sharon fruit, a type of persimmon, are packed with energizing and immune-boosting **antioxidants**, *including* **vitamin C, beta-carotene, lycopene, lutein and zeaxanthin**. *A good source of* **dietary fibre** *and minerals* **magnesium, manganese, potassium, iron and calcium**, *they are beneficial for* **heart health** *and encourage* **detoxification** *and elimination of waste.*

Nutritional analysis per serving: *Calories 46kcal • Protein 0.6g • Carbohydrates 10.7g • Fat 0.1g (of which saturates 0g)*

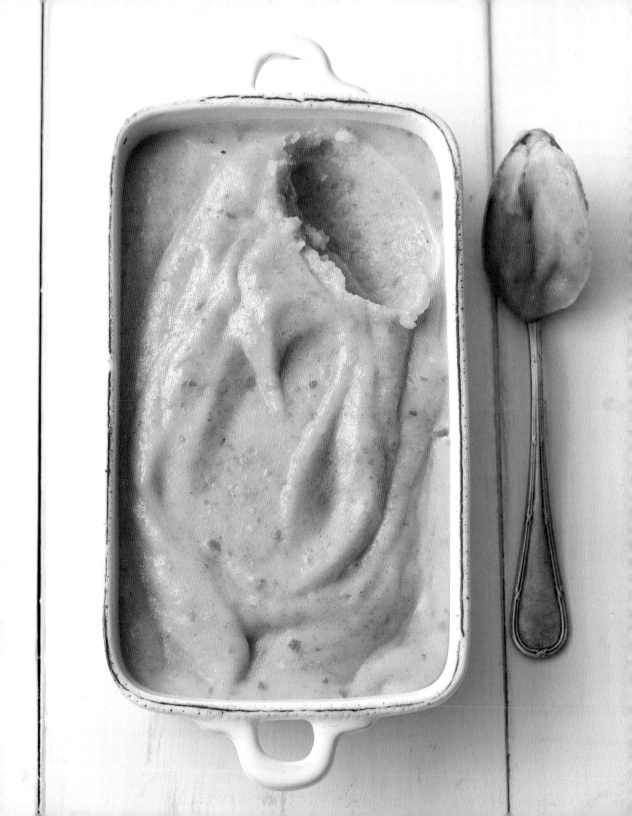

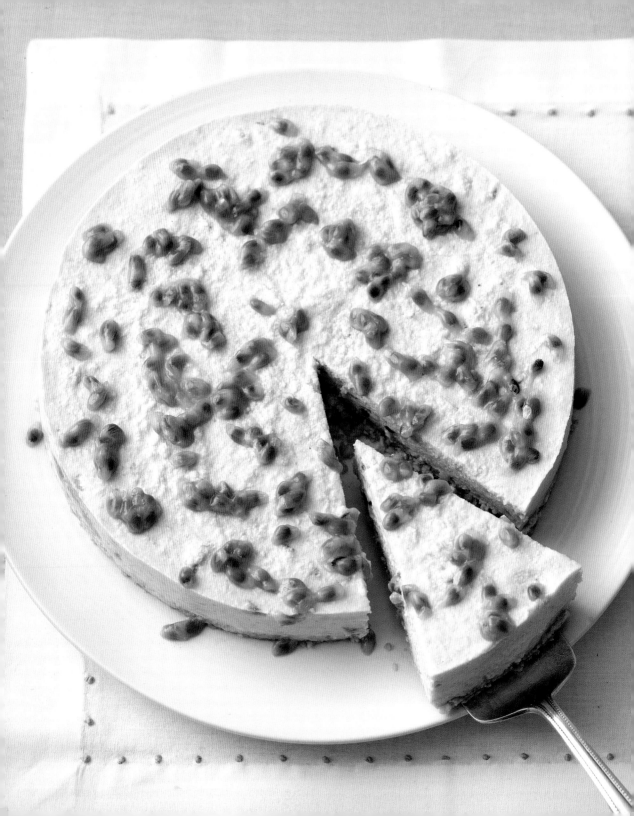

< passion fruit & orange cheesecake

A tropical-flavoured base, topped with a creamy citrus and passion fruit filling, creates this delicious fuss-free dessert – ideal for entertaining or for a special treat. It is low in sugar, yet packed with nutrients and protein.

PREPARATION TIME: *20 minutes, plus 2 hours freezing time and 1 hour defrosting time* ● **STORAGE**: *will keep in the fridge for up to 3 days. Can be frozen for up to 1 month* ● **SERVES**: *10–12*

BASE: 125g/4½oz/heaped ¾ cup cashew nuts ● 80g/3oz/1 cup desiccated coconut ● pinch sea salt ● 2 tbsp yacon syrup ● 3 tbsp lemon juice ● 1 tbsp coconut butter, melted

FILLING: 250g/9oz/1⅔ cups cashew nuts ● 75g/3oz/½ cup coconut butter ● juice of ½ lemon ● zest of 2 oranges ● juice of 4 oranges, about 300ml/10½fl oz/1¼ cups ● pinch sea salt ● 1 tsp vanilla extract ● 3 tbsp xylitol ● 8 passion fruit

1 Make the base by grinding the nuts and coconut in a blender until finely chopped. Stir in the remaining ingredients, adding a little water, if needed, to bind the dough. Press firmly into the base of a 20cm/8in springform cake tin. Freeze while you make the filling.
2 Blend all the remaining ingredients, except the passion fruit, in a blender until smooth. Scoop the pulp from the passion fruit and swirl half of it into the filling. Pour the mixture over the base and freeze for 2 hours until set.
3 Remove the cheesecake from the tin and transfer to the fridge. Allow to defrost for 1 hour before serving.
4 Top with the remaining passion fruit pulp to serve.

HEALTH BENEFITS
*Passion fruit are packed with **antioxidants**, particularly **vitamin C, vitamin A, and phenolic and flavonoid compounds**, to support **immune health** and protect against certain forms of **cancer**. The seeds are a good source of **fibre**, useful for regulating bowel function.*

Nutritional analysis per serving (for 10): *Calories 309kcal ● Protein 6.3g ● Carbohydrates 13.7g ● Fat 26.5g (of which saturates 12.8g)*

superfood candies >

Scrummy little treats that are perfect for when you get the munchies, and a great healthy alternative to sweets and chocolate bars. While these include a range of superfoods, you can vary the ingredients according to taste.

SOAKING TIME: *10 minutes* • **PREPARATION TIME:** *20 minutes* • **STORAGE:** *will keep in the fridge for up to 3–4 days* • **MAKES**: *16 candies*

125g/4¼oz/1¼ cups pecan nuts • 1 tbsp lucuma powder • 1 tbsp maca powder • 4 tbsp raw cacao powder • 2 tbsp xylitol • 1 tbsp flower pollen granules • 60g/2¼oz/½ cup goji berries (soaked for 10 minutes, then drained) • 10 pitted dates (soaked for 10 minutes, then drained) • 3 tbsp coconut butter, melted • desiccated coconut, for rolling

1 Place the pecans, lucuma powder, maca powder, cacao powder and xylitol in a blender or food processor and process to form a fine powder. Place in a bowl with the flower pollen.
2 Place the dried fruit and coconut butter in the blender or food processor and process to form a sticky paste – still keeping some texture. Knead into the dry ingredients to form a stiff dough.
3 Form into balls, then roll in the desiccated coconut.

HEALTH BENEFITS
*Goji berries are an extremely nutrient-dense, rich fruit, bursting with **antioxidants, amino acids, trace minerals** and energising **B vitamins**. They are also rich in **polysaccharides** and traditionally regarded as a longevity- and immune-supporting food. Being rich in the antioxidants **zeaxanthin and lutein**, they are also useful for **healthy vision**.*

Nutritional analysis per candy: *Calories 135kcal • Protein 2.5g • Carbohydrates 11.8g • Fat 8.7g (of which saturates 3.1g)*

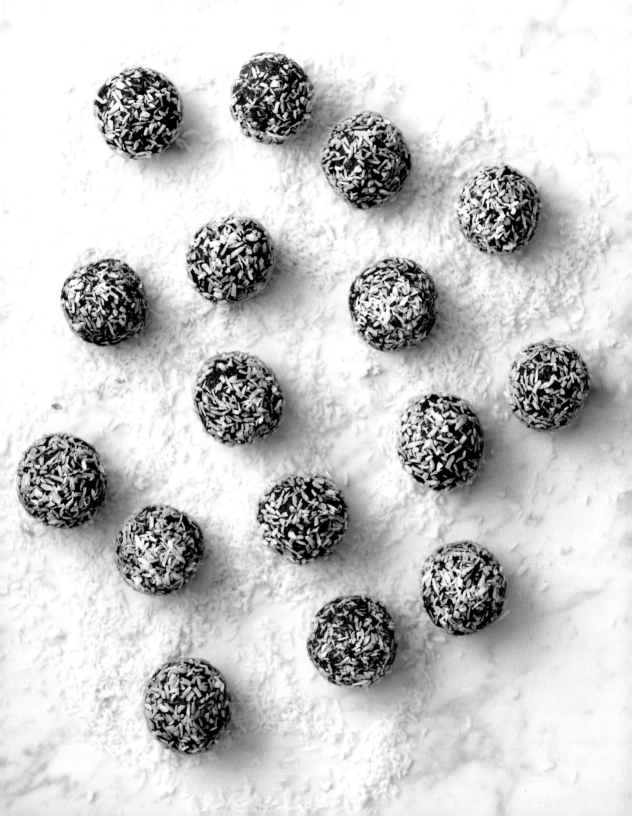

index